HEART ATTACKS – PREVENT AND SURVIVE

DR TOM SMITH spent six years in general practice and seven years in medical research before taking up writing full-time in 1977. He writes regularly for medical journals and magazines and has a weekly column in the *Bradford Telegraph and Argus*. He is the author of *Living with High Blood Pressure, Coping with Strokes, Coping with Bronchitis and Emphysema* and *Living with Alzheimer's Disease* (all Sheldon Press). He still does some general practice in South West Scotland. He is married with two married children and four grandchildren.

Overcoming Common Problems Series

For a full list of titles please contact
Sheldon Press, Marylebone Road, London NW1 4DU

Antioxidants
Dr Robert Youngson

The Assertiveness Workbook
Joanna Gutmann

Beating the Comfort Trap
Dr Windy Dryden and Jack Gordon

Body Language
Allan Pease

Body Language in Relationships
David Cohen

Calm Down
Dr Paul Hauck

Cancer – A Family Affair
Neville Shone

The Cancer Guide for Men
Helen Beare and Neil Priddy

The Candida Diet Book
Karen Brody

Caring for Your Elderly Parent
Julia Burton-Jones

Cider Vinegar
Margaret Hills

Comfort for Depression
Janet Horwood

Considering Adoption?
Sarah Biggs

Coping Successfully with Hay Fever
Dr Robert Youngson

Coping Successfully with Pain
Neville Shone

Coping Successfully with Panic Attacks
Shirley Trickett

Coping Successfully with PMS
Karen Evennett

Coping Successfully with Prostate Problems
Rosy Reynolds

Coping Successfully with RSI
Maggie Black and Penny Gray

Coping Successfully with Your Hiatus Hernia
Dr Tom Smith

Coping Successfully with Your Irritable Bladder
Dr Jennifer Hunt

Coping Successfully with Your Irritable Bowel
Rosemary Nicol

Coping When Your Child Has Special Needs
Suzanne Askham

Coping with Anxiety and Depression
Shirley Trickett

Coping with Blushing
Dr Robert Edelmann

Coping with Bronchitis and Emphysema
Dr Tom Smith

Coping with Candida
Shirley Trickett

Coping with Chronic Fatigue
Trudie Chalder

Coping with Coeliac Disease
Karen Brody

Coping with Cystitis
Caroline Clayton

Coping with Depression and Elation
Dr Patrick McKeon

Coping with Eczema
Dr Robert Youngson

Coping with Endometriosis
Jo Mears

Coping with Epilepsy
Fiona Marshall and
Dr Pamela Crawford

Coping with Fibroids
Mary-Claire Mason

Coping with Gallstones
Dr Joan Gomez

Coping with Headaches and Migraine
Shirley Trickett

Coping with a Hernia
Dr David Delvin

Coping with Long-Term Illness
Barbara Baker

Coping with the Menopause
Janet Horwood

Coping with Psoriasis
Professor Ronald Marks

Coping with Rheumatism and Arthritis
Dr Robert Youngson

Overcoming Common Problems Series

Overcoming Common Problems Series

Overcoming Common Problems

Heart Attacks - Prevent and Survive

Dr Tom Smith

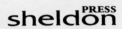

First published in Great Britain in 1990
Sheldon Press, 1 Marylebone Road, London NW1 4DU

Revised and updated 1995, 2000

© Dr Tom Smith 1990, 1995, 2000

New edition 2000
Second impression 2002

Illustrations by Alasdair J. D. Smith

British Library Cataloguing-in-Publication Data

A catalogue record for this book is available from the British Library

ISBN 0–85969–840–8

Typeset by Deltatype Limited, Birkenhead, Merseyside
Printed in Great Britain by Biddles Ltd
www.biddles.co.uk

Contents

Introduction

The greatest cause of early death in the developed world, and particularly in the United Kingdom, is 'heart attack'. One person in three in England and Wales, and almost one in two in Scotland and Northern Ireland, dies from a heart attack, often before retirement age.

Yet we can all do something to lower our risk of early death. This book explains how we can help ourselves, whether we are still fit and healthy, or already have a heart or circulation problem.

It also explains the background to common heart conditions and the new developments in their investigation and treatment. It replaces the natural fear of heart disease with understanding, which is in itself a major step towards better health.

The book does have a strong and simple theme. There are three main, proven causes of heart attacks: cigarette smoking, high blood pressure, and high levels of cholesterol in the blood. If we can keep all three under control, then we will hugely improve our chances of living to a happy, productive and worthwhile old age. Everything else, such as heredity, stress levels, obesity, lack of exercise and even alcohol consumption, although important for general health, is secondary to these three in terms of heart attacks.

We are bombarded today with all sorts of advice on keeping the heart healthy. We hear almost daily about 'risk factors', 'cures' and other 'treatments', some based on fact, but much based on conjecture and even on food fads. I have tried to sort out the wheat from the chaff.

This book, therefore, is partly a guide to sensible living for your heart's sake. It spells out the risks we all face, how to reduce them, and the evidence that proves we are on the right track.

However, it also recognizes that many people already have 'heart' symptoms. You may have angina. The book describes how to recognize that you have a problem, and how it will be investigated and treated. It explains terms such as angina, coronary thrombosis and myocardial infarction, and takes the fear out of coronary care units.

You, or your spouse, may already have had a heart attack. If so,

1

you should find this book very helpful. A heart attack isn't the end of the world – and there are many ways in which you can help yourself or your partner to recover from it, and to prevent further attacks. These are all explained in the later chapters.

One of the most confusing aspects of heart disease is diet. We are bombarded with propaganda on 'healthy' eating for the heart. The 'butter versus margarine', 'red meat versus poultry and fish', 'high fibre versus sugar' and 'fish oils, polyunsaturates and monounsaturates' debates are explored. What is not in the book is a detailed diet sheet – and the reason for its omission is made clear.

The book ends with an appendix on the current prescription drugs for heart disease. Many heart patients take several different tablets and capsules a day, without knowing what they are for. Knowing why you are taking a particular drug can help when a doctor unknown to you may have to take charge in an emergency. Understanding your treatment is as important as understanding your illness.

One aim of the book is to take the pain out of changing your, or your partner's lifestyle towards a healthier heart. It concentrates on the benefits, the good things, about the new way to live – the little things that make it a pleasure to change, rather than a drudge. It's not difficult to change your eating habits, if what you are turning to is better and tastier. Or to stop smoking, if you add up all the benefits – and they are almost countless! Or to start to make yourself physically fit again – if it is *fun!*

Most people who would choose to buy this book will do so because they, or a close relative, already have a heart complaint. However, it should interest *any* adult. The heart attack rates start to climb for apparently healthy men from the early 40s onwards, and for women in the late 50s. A first heart attack often comes out of the blue: reading this book, and taking the steps it recommends, may postpone it or even prevent it altogether.

1
Heart deaths –
the scale of the problem

In Britain, diseases of the heart and circulation claim 300,000 lives every year. They far outnumber deaths from any other cause, and one-third of the deaths are in people who have not yet reached 65.

'Heart attacks', from coronary heart disease, are the cause of most of these early deaths, and greatly reduce the enjoyment of life in many survivors.

Don't, however, let this gloomy start put you off reading further. For this book is optimistic. Although heart attacks are the great risk of our time – the chances of the average person contracting AIDS, for example, are vanishingly small, compared with the heart attack risk – there is plenty of evidence that most people can take successful, practical and even enjoyable steps to avoid them.

You may think that you have heard all this before, that this is one of those books that urges you to exercise, to go on a healthy diet, and to make life generally miserable for yourself. And that it will be as confusing as all the others – because it offers no proof that what it advises will do any good.

Not so. Because it presents the facts, drawn from a whole series of surveys and trials of tens of thousands of people from all over the world. The conclusions are, at last, beyond argument.

If you are sceptical about this, it is understandable. The medical profession, nutritionists and the food industry were rightly blamed for putting out confusing messages in the past. Now we are getting it right. People are no longer exhorted to 'go to work on an egg', or to 'drink a pint of milk a day'. We know much more about good nutrition and the other habits that make for better health. All that is needed is to persuade the public that we have it right this time.

That is why this chapter is devoted to the evidence – the studies that prove just why people have heart attacks, and how they can be avoided. It should convince the most sceptic – and that is the first step to making the life changes that are needed. It is no use deciding to change your lifestyle if you are not fully convinced of the reason for doing so: the change will be shortlived. Read this first chapter, and be convinced: the rest of the book will help you put your newfound resolve into practice.

Wartime Norway – the 'natural experiment'

Before the Second World War, the Norwegians enjoyed a very high standard of living. In particular, they ate well. They also had a very high death rate from heart attacks. The Nazi occupation was very unpleasant, but it did have its silver lining.

From 1940 onwards, the Norwegians were cut off from their sources of tobacco. Many were forced by the occupying Nazis into more physically active jobs. Their diet changed: their milk, beef and cheeses were exported to Germany, so that they had to rely much more on fish for their main food. They lost weight, and their blood pressures fell. This was at a time, of course, of the most immense stress. For four years, the average Norwegian lived constantly with fear and anxiety such as most of us can hardly imagine.

From 1941 onwards, however, the number of Norwegian deaths from heart attacks and circulation disorders fell steeply. This fall in heart deaths coincided with an even steeper drop in the numbers of hospital patients who had thrombosis (blood clots) after operations.

Yet only two years after the war ended, with the return to abundant food and cigarettes, despite the fall in stress, the heart attack rates rose again to the prewar levels.

The Norwegian 'natural experiment', which was probably mirrored in other occupied European countries, such as the Netherlands, has two lessons for us in the early 2000s. The first is that, even when the answers are staring us in the face, it takes far too long for people to accept the truth, if it means a radical re-approach to life. It took a further 30 years for the medical profession to fully accept the facts on diet, smoking, exercise and heart disease – and the average person either still has doubts about them or does not care. That is, until he or she is faced with his or her own mortality.

The second and more important lesson is that it takes only a short time – less than a year – for such a change to make a substantial improvement in our chances of avoiding an early 'heart' death.

The Norwegian experience was only one example of how populations can improve their chances of avoiding heart attacks. Since the 1950s a whole series of studies have confirmed the risks and how to lower them.

The need for proof

Why should these studies have been necessary? The plain fact is that the medical profession had no real idea what was causing so many people to die from heart trouble. The very word 'coronary thrombosis', so commonplace today, was not coined until the 1920s. This was when the pathologists finally proved that many 'heart' deaths were due to a blockage (a clot, or thrombosis) in the blood vessels, the coronary arteries, that supply the heart muscle with its oxygen and energy. There is more about that in Chapter 2.

Victorian doctors, to judge from their records, saw much less heart disease than their modern counterparts. Of course, many Victorians died young, from infections and other diseases of poverty, so that they did not reach the 'coronary' age group. Enough of them survived into old age, however, to have made heart attacks relatively common, if they had had the susceptibility to heart disease that we have now.

So something has changed, greatly to the disadvantage of our hearts, in the last 100 years or so. All sorts of possibilities were put forward by the medical pundits of the 1950s. They included our new-found affluence – which was linked with our softer living, the richer diet, the lack of exercise. Other suggestions were increased stress – although when studied in detail, it hardly seemed possible that the stresses of living are worse now for the average person than they were in the desperate social conditions of the last century.

There were even suggestions that the main risk of heart disease was inherited. Families in which most of the men and women died early from heart attacks were cited as proof that there were genetic factors predisposing to them. The discovery that some of these families had had levels of fat in their blood – *quite unrelated to their diet* – seemed to confirm this.

Why had these families only now been recognized? The glib answer was that in past generations they had also been more susceptible than others to infections, and that their deaths had been lost in the mass of other early deaths. However, it became obvious that inheritance accounts for only a small proportion of deaths from heart attacks. Heart attacks hit most families indiscriminately. There had to be environmental factors, as well as inheritance, that predisposed to an attack. If they could be found, they might be reversed. The same could hardly be said for inheritance, so the search for some other cause was at least more likely to produce practical results!

The lack of knowledge of the true causes of heart attack did not prevent governments from promoting campaigns on health that, in retrospect, were much more to do with maintaining the agricultural economy than with the true care of the people.

In Britain, for example, the need to be self-sufficient in food, which had been so obvious in the Second World War, was all-important. Farms had to be revitalized, and farmers supported at all costs. The dairy, beef and egg producers, in particular, had to be promoted. The 'Eat British beef', 'Drink a pint of milk a day', and 'Go to work on an egg' campaigns were the most intense advertising pressures ever to be put on the people.

Agriculturally, they worked superbly. Farming turned, in only three decades, from the bankrupt, poverty-stricken, labour-intensive disaster of the 1930s, when the British had to import most of their essential foods, to the rich, but subsidized, vast, modernized, intensive factory-based system of today.

As the new farm products hit the markets, and the economy recovered from the war, the diet of the people changed accordingly. 'Quality' foods had never before been so cheap. And as the consumption of animal fats in milk products, eggs and meats rose, the deaths from heart attacks rose in almost exact parallel.

The same pattern was being repeated in other northern European countries, particularly Scandinavia, and in North America. With the end of war, and recovery of the economy, came affluence. And with affluence came the rising tide of heart attacks.

By the late 1950s, the toll of deaths from heart attacks could no longer be ignored. Until then, it has to be admitted, doctors could only pontificate about the possible causes, and the advice people were given about caring for their hearts depended on their doctor's personal judgement (or prejudice).

Another revolution was taking place in health at precisely the same time. The first effective drugs to treat tuberculosis, streptomycin and isoniazid, had been introduced. Throughout the first forty years of this century, tuberculosis was the biggest chronic health problem in Britain. It was treated, in the main, by placing people in long stay sanitoria. Whole hospitals were devoted to tuberculosis.

In the mid-1950s these hospitals closed. Thousands of beds were emptied as the new drugs, and the better social conditions, allowed

TB patients to come home and live again among the community. Doctors who had specialized in tuberculosis had to seek other diseases to treat.

They did not have long to wait. For in only three or four years the 'chest' beds filled up again. The new patients now had chronic bronchitis, and worse still, lung cancer.

There had to be a reason for this sudden swing in the pattern of diseases – and it had to be found in the changing habits of the people. The most obvious was in smoking. Smoking, of course, directly affects the lungs. It puts the most delicate membrane in the body, the sheet of cells lining the lungs, in direct contact with hot, tar-filled smoke and poisonous gases. It has to be damaging.

The timing was right, too. It wasn't until the start of the First World War that the average man started to smoke cigarettes regularly. The women followed, one war later. The great rise in bronchitis and lung cancer figures started one generation earlier in the men – and by 1960, they were both obviously on the upsurge in women. All the models of the two diseases suggested a twenty-year gap between the start of smoking and their onset. Cigarette smoking had to be one of the suspect causes.

The concern about smoking spilled over into the field of the physicians who treated the other organ in the chest, the heart. Their specialty was undergoing a revolution, too. Medical students in the 1950s learned much more about rheumatic heart disease – a condition of the heart valves that followed rheumatic fever in childhood – than about coronary disease and heart attacks. In every hospital general medical ward, there were two or three young adults, men and women, dying slowly of rheumatic heart failure. They outnumbered the patients recovering from 'heart attacks'.

Today's medical students would be lucky to see a case of rheumatic heart disease in the whole of their student career. Rheumatic fever has virtually disappeared as a childhood disease, mainly because children's health and living conditions are so much better. And when it does occur, it is much more effectively treated, with penicillin and aspirin, so that the heart complications do not arise. (Aspirin is not recommended for children under twelve years old, except in rheumatic fever and some other specialist areas, such as arthritis.)

At the same time as the 'chest' beds were filling up with bronchitis and lung cancer cases, the occupants of the 'heart' beds were changing, too. Instead of having rheumatic heart disease, they had quite a different condition – atherosclerosis (dealt with in detail in Chapter 2): for the moment it is enough to know that it is the disease that lies behind heart attacks and angina pectoris – the pain in the chest that warns of possible impending heart attack.

So, in the 1950s the medical profession was faced with a rapidly rising number of cases of heart and lung disease. The problem was not just one of treatment; by the time patients reached the wards with lung cancers, chronic bronchitis and the aftermath of heart attacks, most were already destined for poor health and an early death. What was urgently needed was some way to stop the toll – and that meant *prevention*.

Diseases can only be prevented if the causes are known and addressed. To find them, the clinicians, who take care of individual patients, had to turn to the epidemiologists, who study the pattern of diseases and lifestyles in populations. Happily, in the 1950s the western world was very well served by excellent epidemiologists who knew exactly what to do.

Epidemiology – the burden of proof

Suggesting that a particular pattern of behaviour, such as diet or smoking, may lead to a disease, is one thing. *Proving* that it does is quite another. Take the Norwegian evidence mentioned above. Well after the war was over, people looked at statistics gathered before, during and just after the war years and analysed them in retrospect. The aim was to discover links, if any, between behaviour or environment and eventually health.

Scientifically, this type of analysis can be used as a pointer to further, planned studies, but cannot be regarded as proof of cause and effect. There are too many unidentifiable variables which may cause bias in the results. In Norway, too many aspects of life changed at the same time to be able to judge the relative importance of one over another.

For example, suppose that smoking has a much more powerful effect than a change in diet. Stopping smoking may have been so beneficial to the Norwegians that a less severe, but still bad, effect on diet (say, that switching from beef to fish was actually bad) would have been overlooked. On the other hand the extra stress of wartime life may have actually been very good for the heart, and have more than compensated for a possible bad effect, however unlikely, of stopping smoking.

The only way to sort out these problems is to perform large-scale *prospective* studies of whole populations. The sample size has to be so large that it will show any differences in health risk between people with different backgrounds and lifestyles. Obviously preventive studies have to start when the subjects are still in normal health, and the researchers have to keep in close contact with them all, over many years, so that any changes in their health, and causes of death, can be recorded.

The problems inherent in such studies should not be underestimated. It means following several thousand people, even tens of thousands, in some studies, in a population, chosen at random, in their early, fit years. They are then watched for the rest of their lives. The researchers are people, too, so those who set up the programmes will probably not see their completion.

The people under survey have to submit themselves to extensive invasion of their lives, knowing that the research will not directly benefit themselves, but the generations that will follow. Unless they fall ill, and need medical treatment, they will be expected not to change their lifestyles, and to report any move they may make.

The researchers must take into account every possible aspect of life that may impinge on health. This means thorough investigation, not just of such things as eating, drinking, smoking and exercise habits, but of past personal and family medical problems. It means the physical examination of every subject, from height and weight to pulse rates, blood pressure readings, urine analysis, blood tests and electrocardiograms (ECGs). Social status matters, too. Occupation, marital state, housing and even local climate all come under consideration.

From then on, it is a matter of waiting to see what will happen to the study population. All deaths are reported, and the causes recorded from the doctor's report, preferably from post-mortem examination. In many studies, all reports of survival from heart attack, or the onset of all new cases of angina, are noted, as are deaths and illnesses from all other causes.

The results are worked out using a pre-planned statistical analysis, structured so that the different factors with a potential for causing disease may be taken together and separately. Nothing is left to chance beforehand, because once such a study has started, it is inadmissible, statistically, to alter the analytical or assessment conditions.

All the major studies of heart disease started since the 1950s have followed this pattern. They differ in their details, but their messages have turned out to be the same. The next few pages describe a few of them, to emphasize how solid the proof of the causes of heart attacks has become.

It must be noted here that all the original studies into heart disease concentrated on men. This was largely because, in the 1950s, there were far more male than female heart attack victims, and their heart attacks started at a much younger age. The logic at the time was that if the research concentrated on men, it would lead to much faster results!

Women were thought, at that time, to be largely protected from early heart attacks by the hormones of their menstrual cycle, although the mechanism of this protection was never clearly spelt out. Heart attacks in women will therefore be dealt with in Chapter 8.

The Americans – the Framingham study

The first of the studies, and probably the best known to doctors, was the Framingham study. Researchers persuaded over 5,000 middle-aged men in a small East Coast American town to allow their lives to be studied until they died. From the 1940s onwards the cause of every death of a Framinghamian has been recorded and related to his lifestyle and health on entry to the study. The study subjects were even followed if they moved away from the town – surprisingly few of them have been lost to the researchers' scrutiny.

The facts about the Framingham population are now in the millions. From the study around 3,500 people have now died, so that the conclusions drawn from them are unarguable. Smokers died several years before non-smokers, from heart disease, as well as from lung diseases such as cancer and bronchitis. Men with uncontrolled high blood pressure died early, from strokes and heart attacks. Diabetics also tended to have heart and circulation disorders that shortened their lives.

What surprised the doctors most, however, was the very close relationship between death from heart attacks and the level of fat, and particularly cholesterol, in the blood. A higher than average cholesterol level put the men at particularly high risk of a 'coronary' death, a risk that was multiplied many-fold if it was linked with cigarette smoking, and even more so if it was also linked with high blood pressure. I will deal extensively with cholesterol in Chapter 3.

Could control of these three factors, it was asked, be the answer to the heart disease pandemic that was killing half of the population of the United States? Did they apply equally to people in other countries? More crucially, would altering them, by persuading whole populations to change their habits, make any difference to the numbers of people who were dying before their time?

The Finnish experience

One country, Finland, took on the challenge. The medical authorities there had known for years that one province, North Karelia, had had very high rates of illness and death from heart disease. Most North Karelians were dairy farmers, living mainly on beef and dairy products. Their blood cholesterol levels, which relate directly to animal fat consumption, were much higher than those in other Finns.

The Finnish government embarked on a massive public health programme, aiming to change the diet away from their milk and beef bias and towards vegetable fibre and fish. Within two to three years, the coronary rates were already beginning to improve. Now the North Karelians are well down the league table of heart attack victims.

In Britain now

Meanwhile, the British were aware of their own problem – about a century late. As long ago as 1871, a Dr Haviland wrote about the big differences in numbers of deaths from 'heart disease and dropsy' (the fluid swelling that usually denotes heart failure) in the various regions of England and Wales. Dr Haviland drew a line from the Severn Estuary to the Wash: to the north the people were especially prone to heart disease. To the south of the line, they appeared to be protected against it.

That line, in fact, neatly divided the prosperous from the poor, but the cause of the difference was not so simple. The difference was still there, 100 years later. It took the British Regional Heart Study, conducted throughout the last ten years, to begin to explain it.

This study, which started in January 1978, followed the progress of 7,735 men aged 40 to 59, selected from the lists of doctors in 24 towns in England, Wales and Scotland. Some had been born in their town, some had moved there from elsewhere in Britain, and some were immigrants. Most were apparently healthy when they were picked for the study: some already had signs of heart disease.

After six and a half years, 373 of the men had had heart attacks, just over a third of which were fatal. Men living in the south of England had the fewest attacks: those living in Scotland had the most – twice as many as the southern English residents. There was a 'gradient' of risk, so that each district had a higher heart attack rate than its neighbour to the immediate south, and the gradient was the same for people who had moved into the district, whether British-born or international immigrant. The 'Haviland line' of 1871 still exists today.

The figures for people who had moved from one district to another argued against the inheritance of a 'heart attack risk'. They also suggest that poorer living standards and nutrition in infancy and childhood, features connected with more northern towns, did *not* predict future heart attacks.

The only possible explanation for the difference is that men in a particular geographical zone share a common environment in their adult life that shapes their risk of heart disease. The authors of the Heart Study Report, Professor A. G. Shaper and his colleagues, of the Royal Free Hospital, London, made their conclusions clear in their *Lancet* report in 1989.

Some of the differences may be put down to water hardness (the softer the water, the higher the heart attack rate), rainfall, and temperature. The colder the temperature and the wetter the weather, the higher was the risk of heart attack. Wet Wales, for example, had higher heart attack rates than drier East Anglia on the same latitude.

These differences are small, however, compared to personal characteristics such as high blood pressure, cigarette smoking and social class. The lower on the social ladder, the more chance there is of a heart attack – a conclusion that may surprise people who think of heart attacks as the 'executive's' disease.

Even then, the answers are not simple. Professor Michael Oliver, who was at the University of Edinburgh and is now in London, has worked for years on the reasons for Scotland's unenviable position at the top of the league, worldwide, for heart attack deaths. He points out that not all heavy smoking nations, such as the Japanese, have high heart attack rates. The Japanese do, however, have low blood cholesterol levels, and this has been cited as protecting them against the smoking effect.

That still does not convince Professor Oliver. The southern French, he stresses, not only smoke as much as the Scots, but they also eat plenty of fat and have high blood cholesterol levels. Yet they have *very low* heart attack rates.

According to Professor Oliver, it is not the *amount* of fat we eat, but the *type* of fat, that determines our heart attack risk. His team measured the fat levels in the tissues of Scotsmen and compared them with the levels in Finns, Swedes (whose heart attack rates are low) and in southern Italians.

Linoleic acid

In every case, the level of one particular type of fat stood out as being closely related to heart attack risk. This was linoleic acid, a 'polyunsaturated' fat which is eaten in cereals and vegetable oils such as olive oil. (The differences between 'unsaturated' and 'saturated' fats will be explained in detail in Chapter 3.) In every study, populations with *low* levels of linoleic acid in the fatty tissues, such as the Scots and Finns, had *high* heart attack rates. In the Mediterranean subjects, with high linoleic acid levels, the heart attack rates were low, even when they smoked heavily.

The linoleic acid was not the only difference. The Mediterranean diet provided a high intake of fish, citrus fruits and green vegetables, all of which, Professor Oliver stressed, help to prevent the blood clotting that is the essential first step in a heart attack.

Not surprisingly, Professor Oliver exhorts everyone to eat as most people do along the Mediterranean shores. Stopping smoking will also help, but those who cannot or will not should make a special effort to eat healthily. They will not be protected against the other diseases caused by smoking, such as bronchitis, emphysema and lung cancer, but they may reduce their heart attack risk.

Interestingly, smoking and fat levels may themselves be connected, at least in the United Kingdom. The Edinburgh research showed that coronary-prone people and those who already have heart attacks do not eat much food that contains linoleic acid. Cigarette smokers, it was found, were even more selective in their choice of food: they had real *dislikes* for foods containing the 'protective' fats. The more cigarettes they smoked, the less linoleic acid they had in their tissues. The smokers also consumed less fish and less vegetable fibre than the non-smokers.

This difference did not depend on social class, but it was linked to alcohol intake; the smokers drank more than the non-smokers. Similar results were reported from South Wales, where the Caerphilly Heart Disease Study, involving 493 middle-aged men, reported in 1984 that smokers ate less vegetable fibre and more total fat than non-smokers.

Professor Oliver suggested that cigarette smoking so injures the *taste buds* that food containing the protective vegetable fats and oils somehow tastes less pleasant, so that it is rejected, either consciously or subconsciously. The fact that smokers add much more salt than usual to their food suggests that the habit alters – some would say poisons – the taste system.

Fibrinogen – the 'clotting protein'

There are ways other than its effects on blood fats in which smoking raises the risk of a heart attack. Dr Tom Meade and his team at the Northwick Park Hospital, London, in a study involving 2,023 men, found a very close relationship between smoking and levels of a protein called fibrinogen in the blood.

The more cigarettes they smoked, the higher were the men's fibrinogen levels. This is bad news, because fibrinogen is used naturally to promote clotting of blood – it is one of the ways the body stops bleeding after an injury. Unfortunately, when fibrinogen levels rise too high, the blood can clot *too easily* in places where clotting can be dangerous – as in the coronary arteries in the heart. This is one of the main causes of heart attacks. Several studies have proved that the blood in 'coronary' patients contains more fibrinogen than normal.

Fibrinogen levels cannot be changed much by altering diet: some people inherit a tendency to raised fibrinogen, but inheritance plays a small part. Smoking is by far the commonest and easiest way to raise our fibrinogen levels – and when we stop the habit, they return quickly to normal. So stopping smoking benefits the potential heart attack victim, which in our society includes us all, in several ways.

The MRFIT 'screenees'

Persuasive as they are, none of the studies described so far can compare with the results from the most complicated trial of all – the MRFIT study. This was set up in the United States to test if it were possible to reduce the numbers of coronary attacks in middle-aged men at high risk. Called the *M*ultiple *R*isk *F*actor *I*ntervention *T*rial (hence MRFIT), it screened 361,662 men aged between 35 and 57 over two years from 1973.

The men's birthdate, social security number (to establish social and occupational status), smoking habit, blood pressure and blood cholesterol were all noted at entry to MRFIT, and later related to their subsequent causes of death. By 1982, 7,820 of the men had died, 2,626 from coronary heart disease and 2,365 from cancer. These figures were expected: heart disease and cancer are by far the two most common causes of death in any developed nation.

Half of all the deaths from coronary heart disease were in the men in the top 15 per cent for blood cholesterol level. The higher the blood pressure and the higher the blood cholesterol level, the higher was the risk of a 'heart' death. The cancer deaths were very strongly related to smoking habit, and not at all to blood pressure.

Interestingly, if there was a relationship between the cancer deaths and cholesterol level, it was in the opposite direction to that with heart attacks. There appeared to be *more* cancer in those with very low cholesterol levels. One proposed reason for this is that some cancers were already in their early stages in some of the subjects, and that this had already lowered their cholesterol levels at the start of the study. The researchers are still debating this point, which will be examined in more detail in Chapter 3.

MRFIT came to the conclusions that all American men should lower the amount of fat in their food – the suggested source of the cholesterol – and that there should be intensive treatment, with drugs and diet, for anyone with a cholesterol reading in the top 15 per cent, or a moderately raised blood pressure, or both.

So for men, at least, keeping heart attacks at bay definitely depends on three key actions. They are:

- don't smoke
- know your cholesterol level and lower it if it is high
- know your blood pressure, and take steps to reduce it if it is high.

How to do these three things is explained in later chapters.

It's never too late to change

We have established beyond any reasonable doubt that smoking, uncontrolled high blood pressure and high levels of cholesterol in the blood are the three main causes of heart attacks. The smoking can be stopped, the blood pressure can be controlled, and the blood cholesterol level can be reduced. If you are a diabetic, then your extra risk of heart attacks can be reduced by better control of your blood sugar and insulin levels.

So why do so many people ignore the warnings, and continue to expose themselves to the high risk? Perhaps they do not relate what they are bound to have read or seen in press or television to themselves. Heart attacks, they believe, happen to other people, not them. As you are concerned enough to have started reading this book, you are not in that category.

You may, however, be in the other group who feel that they have been doing the wrong things – smoking, overeating, underexercising – for so many years that a change now to a better lifestyle would make no difference. That is a plausible excuse for taking no personal action. It is, however, wrong.

There is plenty of evidence, apart from the Norwegian experience, to show that changing lifestyle, even late in life, can reduce risks of heart attacks. Take smoking as an example. The risk of a heart attack after stopping cigarette smoking – no matter how many were smoked per day and for how many years – returns to the risk in 'never-smokers' within two years. The risk of lung cancer after stopping cigarette smoking, again regardless of numbers smoked, returns to normal after ten years.

For every percentage point that the blood cholesterol level is reduced the risk of heart attack is reduced by 2 per cent. The MRFIT study, which concentrated on exercise, changing eating habits towards lowering cholesterol levels and stopping smoking, led to a 16 per cent fall in cases of angina and heart failure.

Of course, no one is going to live until he or she is 140 – who would want to! But changing to a better lifestyle, even after middle age, offers so much more to all of us. It will greatly increase the chance of enjoying an active, fit life in later years. Even if you already have some symptoms of heart disease, changing your lifestyle can help to prevent it worsening, and can even reverse the disease. Men and women who have been 'cardiac cripples' have been helped to walk and enjoy life again.

Chapter 2 explains what happens in heart disease, and why smoking, fats and high blood pressure affect the heart so badly; once you understand this, it is easier to resolve to control them. You may be surprised how easy it is to lower your own risk of heart attack, and to feel fitter and happier in the process.

2

The heart, the circulation,
and blood

The heart is just a pump. All it does it pump blood around the body. The two chambers of the left side of the heart pump blood rich in oxygen from the lungs to the rest of the body. The two corresponding chambers of the right side of the heart take the oxygen-spent, carbon dioxide-rich blood from the body back to the lungs. In the lungs the blood gives up the carbon dioxide – the waste material from the body's energy-burning processes – to the air, and takes in more oxygen.

These are the bald facts. But there is no human-designed pump that could do the heart's job. No engineer has yet made a pump that acts around 70 times a minute, for upwards of 70 years, all the time maintaining and repairing itself and supplying its own energy and fuel. And not once, in all that time, stopping for a rest.

The secret lies in the special properties of the heart muscle. Try to do with your leg muscles what you take for granted that your heart does. Run on the spot so that each foot touches the ground just a little faster than once a second. Step high as you do it, so that your thighs come up to the horizontal with each step. See how long you can carry on before your legs get tired, and have to rest.

If you are relatively unfit, you may last as long as five minutes. Athletes, of course, can go on for an hour or more. But do it day and night, without stopping to sleep and rest? For years? Impossible for even the greatest marathon runner.

Yet that is what the heart does, day in, day out, all our lives. Most of the time we do not give it a second thought. Of course, that is a good thing: people who are constantly aware of their heartbeat can become neurotic and obsessional about it, and their lives can be ruined. In the early days of heart valve surgery, some valve models gave out a 'ping' with each beat. Their owners could hear it plainly, especially at night, and were often, understandably, upset about it.

Yet we need a happy medium in our relationship with our hearts. The more we understand about how the heart works, the better care we should be able to take of it, and the less frightened we should be when it shows signs of going wrong.

First of all, the heart is all muscle, the myocardium (muscle = myo, heart = cardium). It differs from all other muscles in the body by having an astonishing capacity for rapid recovery after it has been 'fired' by nerve impulses to contract, or 'beat'. Given the signal to contract by a special network of electrical fibres exclusive to it alone, it completes its cycle of shortening and lengthening within a fifth of a second, then has three-fifths or four-fifths of a second to recover before it is asked to beat again.

During that vital resting period, the muscle reorganizes itself so that it can contract again without tiring. In the process of contraction it takes oxygen from the blood. Oxygen is the fuel that converts the heart muscle's store of glucose into the energy needed so that it can beat. In the resting period between beats, each muscle fibre has to take up more oxygen and glucose to repeat the cycle. Without the constant flow of oxygen and glucose from the bloodstream, the heart muscle cannot work. It will first complain, and then die. Give it enough nutrients and oxygen and it will keep going for a lifetime.

How the heart beats

Obviously, the blood supply to the heart muscle has to be special. To beat efficiently, the heart has first to push blood from the upper chambers, called the atria, to the lower and larger chambers, the ventricles. The atria beat first, shifting the blood that has returned from the body or lungs into the ventricles. Once filled and stretched by the incoming blood, the ventricles then beat, pushing the blood out into the lungs and the rest of the body.

Once the contraction is over, the heart relaxes. Valves placed in the outflow vessels – the pulmonary artery (to the lungs) and the aorta (to the rest of the body) – prevent the blood just expelled from the heart from flowing back again into it. Instead, even when the heart is in its state of relaxation, the blood is driven onwards by the tension in the closed valves and in the muscles within the walls of the main blood vessels. Meanwhile, more blood is sucked into the atria as the heart relaxes, and the cycle starts again.

This system means that there are two distinct phases of the heart beat. The first is the contraction that forces the blood out through the open valves: this is called *systole*. The pressure exerted on the blood in this action is called the *systolic pressure*.

19

The second is the phase of relaxation of the heart. This is called *diastole*. The pressure of blood within the body's blood vessels while the heart is relaxing is the *diastolic pressure*. Both the systolic and the diastolic pressures are noted when the blood pressure is taken. The first is a measure of the force of the heart beat, the second of the resistance of the blood vessels to the flow of blood within them. Together, they give the doctor a good idea of the state of the circulation.

Blood pressure is measured in units of millimetres of mercury (mmHg), which corresponds to the height of the column of mercury in the sphygmomanometer – the instrument doctors usually use for taking the blood pressure. A figure of 120–140 mmHg is normal for the systolic pressure, and 70–80 for the diastolic pressure. So a normal pressure would be recorded as 120/80 mmHg. A blood pressure of 150/95 is moderately raised. One of 170/105 or above needs investigation.

High blood pressure can be due to excessive force in the heart beat (raising the systolic pressure), or to narrowing of the small blood vessels in the skin and muscles of the limbs (which raises the diastolic pressure). Usually, there is a combination of both.

Blood pressure is needed, of course, to maintain the blood supply to all the organs and structures of the body. The action of systole distributes the blood onwards, and can be felt in the pulse, say, at the wrist or throat.

The coronary arteries

However, there is one organ that is deprived of any flow of blood during systole – the heart itself. When the heart beats, it shortens to half of the volume it is when relaxed. This compresses the blood vessels within its walls, so that the flow of blood within them, and therefore of blood and glucose, stops momentarily.

Instead, these blood vessels, the coronary arteries, so named because they encircle the upper surface of the heart like a crown, have to fill with blood when the heart is relaxing, in diastole. They originate from openings just at the base of the aorta, so that as the valves close against the backward flow of blood, it is diverted into them. The relaxing myocardium virtually sucks its blood supply deep into itself.

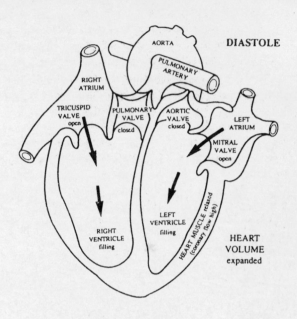

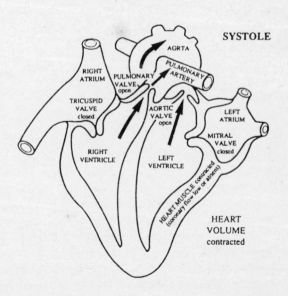

There are two main coronary arteries, one mainly supplying the right, and one the left, sides of the heart. They quickly branch out and dive deep within the heart muscle, so that every part of the heart has its share of oxygen and glucose. In the young and healthy, the coronary arteries are wide, and smooth-lined, so that the blood flows without friction or disturbance through them.

There is even plenty of extra capacity when extra flow is needed. The step-up in energy, for example, when we move from rest to a 100 metre sprint requires shifting the heart rate from 70 to, say, more than 200 beats per minute. This may be combined with a short and sharp rise in blood pressure, perhaps doubling it. At times like these the heart may use up ten to twenty times the amounts of oxygen and glucose used when resting – and must still be able to recover, without tiring, in the very much shorter time between beats.

Athletic training helps the heart to do this very efficiently. The more we use our muscles, the more efficient they become, and the heart muscle is no exception – provided we keep our coronary vessels in a healthy state, too. The coronary arteries are unique in that they widen dramatically in response to the workload they are asked to face. Their walls are marvellously elastic, so that they can take the extra flow of blood through them. There are even extra, unused, channels, called 'collaterals' that will open up to take extra blood if necessary.

Good athletes in training have resting heart rates of 60 or even less, and at top speed may only double or treble them. An unfit, overweight person who runs for a bus may have a pulse racing well above 200 a minute, that will take 20 minutes or more to return to the resting rate between 80 and 90. Add another half as much again to the rise in heart rate and recovery time for a heavy smoker.

The healthy heart

Why the difference? It must be obvious by now that the efficiency of the heart depends on a whole series of properties. It needs blood with the appropriate amounts of oxygen and glucose to fuel the heart muscle. It needs a network of blood vessels, the coronary arteries, which are wide open, free of obstructions, and can expand to take a steep increase in blood flow when needed. It needs a healthy muscle

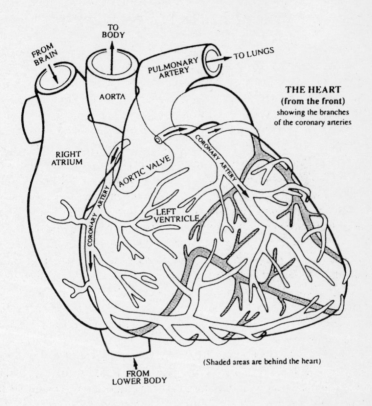

THE HEART
(from the front)
showing the branches
of the coronary arteries

(Shaded areas are behind the heart)

mass, that contracts correctly to time and rhythmically, so that the flow of the circulation from the heart is smooth.

Obviously there are many ways in which we can upset this harmony between the blood, the blood vessels and the heart muscle itself. The act of smoking (we will return to smokers very often in the pages to come) damages the heart muscle in two ways. First, nicotine is a nerve and muscle poison, so that the beat is faster and less efficient. Second, the carbon monoxide inhaled in cigarette smoke both starves the muscle of oxygen and is also a direct muscle poison. This means that the smoker's heart is not only much less efficient, but has much less capacity for recovery when a heart attack threatens.

Of healthy blood vessels

Crucial to the supply of oxygen and glucose to the heart muscle is the state of the coronary arteries that supply them. At birth, their inner lining, the surface in contact with the blood, is smooth, and their walls are muscular and elastic. The blood flows through them smoothly and without eddies or turbulence.

And atheroma

Sadly, as we grow older, this changes. Fatty deposits start to be laid down in the blood vessel walls – the more fat there is in the blood, the more deposits there are. The process starts early. American doctors examining the bodies of young soldiers killed in the Korean War were astonished by the extent of the fatty degeneration in their coronary arteries. It was this work that led to the first real American efforts to prevent heart disease.

In fact, everyone since involved in reducing the numbers of early deaths from heart disease has concentrated on this fatty degeneration in the coronary arteries. The disease has a medical name – atheroma – the ancient Greek word for porridge. Called this because the deposits had the looks and consistency of blobs of porridge, they are crucial to today's understanding about what happens in a heart attack.

Deposits or 'plaques' of atheroma are laid down in the walls of the arteries from childhood onwards. Their numbers and size depend almost entirely on one thing – the levels of cholesterol in the bloodstream. The higher the cholesterol level, the more extensive the atheroma: for people, like some Japanese who live on fish and vegetables, with very low cholesterol levels, there is very little atheroma, and almost no risk of heart attack.

Atheromatous plaques have been extensively analysed. They are made up of a mixture of cholesterol and a combination of fat and protein, known as low density lipoprotein, or LDL. More will be written about this in Chapter 3, but it is enough here to kow that there is a direct relationship between blood levels of LDL-cholesterol and heart attacks. The higher the LDL-cholesterol, the more atheroma appears in the arteries and the higher is the heart attack risk.

There is a simple, mechanical reason for the connection between

24

the two. We now know that most heart attacks are triggered at the site of an atheromatous plaque, where the vessel wall is weakened. The surface of the plaque is roughened, and juts into the stream of blood. This narrowing of the tube within which the blood flows causes eddies and turbulence, with consequent strain on the wall of the blood vessel at precisely the spot where it is weakened.

If that strain becomes too great, the edge of the plaque can lift up with the force of the bloodstream. The blood rushes under the edge, lifting up the plaque to form a flap across the flow, which can be big enough to block it completely. With the flow of blood to the tissues beyond stopped, they will quickly die if they are not relieved – and the heart attack begins.

Angina

Angina, the pain in the chest which some people get with exercise, is explained in a similar way. The coronary arteries in most angina sufferers are so affected by plaques of atheroma that they are much narrower than normal. This means that enough oxygen and glucose is being provided to their heart muscle when they are resting, but as soon as they need to 'step up a gear' for exercise, the narrowed arteries cannot expand enough to cope. The heart runs out of oxygen and glucose and starts to complain. The result is the familiar pain, which will stop with rest as the demand for oxygen and glucose recedes again.

The process can be likened to a car engine. It needs a mixture of air and petrol for the fuel to burn correctly and the energy to be used efficiently. For the heart to work, read oxygen for air, and glucose for petrol. Block the fuel pipe – the coronary arteries – and the machine will not work.

Happily there are ways in which anyone can lower his or her LDL-cholesterol levels, and which directly lower the risk of heart attack. Atheroma is reversible, and its reversibility largely depends on ourselves. We can adopt a lifestyle that has been proved to do so – which means eating healthily, taking exercise and stopping smoking. Over, say, five years, the atheromatous plaques will start to shrink and the arteries will become more flexible again. The secret is to make the change *for the rest of your life*. And, for the small number of people whose atheroma is inherited, there are corrective drugs.

Healthy blood

In addition to a heart that beats efficiently and is in peak condition, and smooth, wide blood vessels, we also need blood that can flow smoothly, without clotting or sticking, through the whole system. Blood is certainly thicker than water, in more than one way. Granted, it is water-based, but it contains within it a 'soup' of substances and cells that makes it much less than free-flowing.

First, there is the *serum*, the fluid in which these substances float. It carries minerals, salts and glucose, all the soluble substances needed for the continuing health of the cells and the waste products for disposal. Then there is the *plasma*. This is the name given to the serum plus a mixture of proteins and fats, mainly derived from our food, essential for all the chemical processes that make life possible. Very fatty plasma is stickier than normal – think of the stickiness left after a fry-up in a pan.

Whole blood is made up of the plasma plus the cells. These include the white cells (*leucocytes*) needed to organize our resistance to infection; '*platelets*', fragments of cells that are much involved in clotting; and the red blood cells (*erythrocytes*) that transport oxygen around the body.

Any fluid engineer would be horrified if asked to design a pump for a closed system of tubing that contained a liquid consisting of such a variety of substances. The difficulties in calculating the various pressures and flow rates are vast. For example, in each segment of the blood – the serum, the plasma and the cells – there are substances which could make the fluid very much more viscous or 'stickier'. When that happens, very much higher pressures are needed to push the fluid through the pipework – and that means more strain on the heart.

Take, for example, the glucose level in the serum. Every cell in the body needs glucose to stay alive: the burning of glucose with oxygen is our main source of energy. So blood must keep its glucose levels within very strict limits. If they fall too low, we become weak and faint as our muscle and brain cells to start to fail. However, if they rise too high, as in diabetes, the blood becomes measurably stickier, and thickens. This is just one of the special problems faced by people with diabetes, who are at particular risk of heart attacks if they do not control their disease very closely.

A rising glucose level, however, is a very minor change compared to what happens when the fat levels rise, or the platelets become 'stickier'. These are changes that can happen to all of us, not just diabetics, and which we can reverse for ourselves. If we let them continue, we raise our risk of heart attack very steeply.

More will be said about this later, but for the moment it is enough to understand that the easiest way to raise the fat levels in the blood is to eat animal (saturated) fats. These are the same fats that are linked with atheroma. Cut down on the animal fat intake, and you will not only help to reverse your atheroma, you will also help to make your blood more fluid – two benefits for the price of one action.

Smoking also features in blood stickiness. Cigarette smoking acts directly upon the platelets – the chemicals absorbed into the blood from the smoke make the platelets stick together. This is the first step towards a blood clot forming in the coronary arteries.

Smoking acts, too, on the muscles in the blood vessel walls themselves. One experiment beloved of medical students in the past was to focus an ophthalmoscope (the instrument used to study the inside of the eye) on a blood vessel in the back of the eye of a non-smoking colleague, then ask him or her to inhale from a cigarette. The effect was dramatic – within seconds the vessel narrows, showing the powerful influence of nicotine. It was enough to put many students off the habit – which was probably the main purpose of the exercise!

Today's equivalent of that experiment is seen in heart departments in every hospital in the country. When patients with angina undergo 'angiography' (the X-ray technique used to study the flow of blood through the coronary arteries) the specialists look not only for the areas of narrowing due to atheroma, but also to the narrowness of the arteries in general.

The X-rays show that in some people the 'resting' diameter of their coronary arteries is much narrower than normal, as if they are stretched out, like elastic. Smokers, for example, inevitably have much narrower coronary arteries than non-smokers. This is because nicotine keeps the blood vessels in a permanent state of increased muscle tone – and the inevitable result is a narrow, thread-like passage, through which it is difficult for the blood to pass.

If that were not enough, smoking has yet another bad effect on the blood. The red cells, which carry the oxygen to the heart muscle, are normally very flexible. They have to be, because they are so wide in one direction. Shaped like thick discs with dimples in their centres (something like a quoit with a filled-in centre), they have to be flexible enough to fold up into tube-like shapes to pass through the smallest blood vessels, the capillaries. The poisons circulating in the blood-streams of smokers make the red cells much less flexible: they stiffen into their rigid, flat disc-like shape.

This not only slows down the progress of the cells through the circulation, it can even help to block the smallest vessels, so that there are many tiny clots, seen only under the microscope, that are constantly putting the delicate tissues of the heart and other organs at risk.

The most extreme form of reaction to smoking in the circulation is Buerger's disease, in which the blood vessels in the legs thicken and 'silt' up. If sufferers do not stop smoking, then most have to have one or two amputations. If they stop, the circulation returns to normal, and they can walk again. It is some testament to the power of tobacco that I have had to care for two patients with Buerger's disease in my time in general practice. Both refused to stop smoking, both had to have both legs amputated, and both eventually died from heart attacks.

Special problems – high blood pressure and diabetes

Two groups of people have a higher than average chance of having a heart attack – those with high blood pressure, and diabetics.

High blood pressure

High blood pressure is, put simply, a state in which the heart is exerting itself more forcefully than needed. This stems from one of two problems. Either the heart beat is too forceful, in which case the systolic pressure is very high, or the small blood vessels in the arms and legs are too narrow, which pushes up the resistance to flow within them, and therefore the diastolic pressure. In most cases of high blood pressure, both are raised.

High blood pressure is a vicious circle: as the pressure rises, the walls of the blood vessels thicken to cope with the strain. This narrows the tubes in which the blood flows even further, which in turn raises the pressure even more. The coronary arteries are no different from the rest: in high blood pressure they narrow like the others, and any narrowing must make them more likely to block if they are also affected by atheroma.

Over years, untreated high blood pressure causes the muscle of the heart to thicken and the heart to enlarge. This produces an extra demand for blood supply and oxygen that eventually cannot be fulfilled through the narrowed coronary arteries. The problem is that while this is happening, high blood pressure sufferers may have no symptoms, and no inkling of their problem. For some the only sign of the rise in pressure is a morning headache, but for most even that is absent. Their first symptoms may be their first heart attack or stroke.

The good news for high blood pressure sufferers is that there are now excellent medical treatments for it that will bring the pressure down to normal levels. This not only reverses the change in the blood vessels, but will also reduce the chances of a heart attack.

Even better news is that most general practitioners now have 'well woman' and 'well man' clinics, one purpose of which is to identify everyone with high blood pressure early. Once diagnosed, it can be treated, and the complications prevented. Everyone over 40 should have their pressures checked; that alone would greatly reduce the numbers of deaths in all developed countries from heart attacks and strokes.

Diabetes

Diabetes is also a matter of good control. The diabetic is at several disadvantages where heart disease is concerned. Diabetics have trouble in getting glucose to where it is needed – the tisues and muscles. For one reason or another, they lack the hormone insulin which shifts the glucose out of the bloodstream into tissues. This means that in untreated or poorly controlled diabetes, the glucose levels in the blood are very high. This not only leads to a sluggish blood flow through the smaller blood vessels, as explained earlier, but it also disturbs the way the body fats are used.

The result is that most diabetics have very high LDL-cholesterol levels in the blood, and that leads to a state of atheroma that is much more severe than normal. So diabetics not only have to control their glucose levels very carefully, by using insulin and watching what they eat, they also have to take particular care of their fat levels. Over and above that, however, we now know that too much insulin can also do them harm. It helps to cause problems in the smallest blood vessels in the kidneys, eyes and skin.

29

Fortunately for all diabetics, there has been real progress in the treatment of the disease in the last ten years. Probably the biggest step forward has been the switch to a high fibre, low fat and low protein diet. This, along with eating many small meals a day, and taking three or four smaller, instead of one or two larger, insulin doses a day, has led to much better control of glucose and insulin levels. That is already reducing the heart attack rates in diabetics regularly attending clinics (those who fall by the wayside and let their control slip do not do so well).

Another big step forward for diabetics is the insulin 'pen'. This springloaded device with a special needle is so much easier, more accurate and less painful to use than the old needle-and-syringe systems that it should be offered to every insulin-using diabetic. It is especially useful for the teenage diabetic, who finds it less embarrassing than syringes, and that it gives him or her much more freedom to live a normal life. It is crucial that good control habits are learned at an early age, because it is at this time that the seed of later trouble in the heart and blood vessels are sown.

Bringing it all together

The message of this chapter is clear. We know a great deal about the problems that underlie most heart attacks.

One is the way we eat – the more fat that is circulating around the body, the higher the risk of heart attack. We can all do something about that.

One is smoking. Smoking raises heart attack risks in several ways. We can do something about that, too.

High blood pressure and diabetes also raise the heart attack risk; both conditions are eminently controllable, and the degree of control largely depends on the sufferers themselves. Lack of exercise is yet another promoter of heart attacks – we can do something about that, too.

Two subjects not mentioned so far, yet popularly connected with heart attacks, are alcohol and stress. It is difficult to link them so directly with higher heart attack risk, but they deserve consideration. Certainly we can all do something about our alcohol consumption and the way we deal with stress.

All these subjects will be covered in the next three chapters, in which the emphasis will be on practical ways to change from a high risk to a low risk lifestyle. We all can do it: we owe it to ourselves and to our families and friends. In one week following the influenza epidemic in the winter of 1989–90 I lost five friends, one a woman, and four men. The youngest was 46, the oldest 61. All died from heart attacks after bouts of influenza.

All were heavy smokers and had eaten, all their lives, not wisely, but too well. It was not the 'flu that killed them – but the fact that the virus pushed them over the knife edge that they had created for themselves.

Influenza was the last straw for them: it had put too much stress on their hearts. Four of them had had the warnings: a mild angina in three, a small previous heart attack in one; but they had all lived what were outwardly normal lives until their sudden, final collapse. For the fifth, the fatal attack came completely out of the blue.

I am sure that all of them would still be alive and with their families today if they had only lived a little differently. It would not have taken much – just a little concern, and respect, for their own bodies. The next chapters suggest how they might have made it through that fatal winter, and laughed at the influenza virus. People cannot avoid catching influenza, but they can try to ensure that it does not put their lives at risk.

3

Cholesterol – facts and fancies, fats and fish

Everyone living in any developed country must have heard about cholesterol. The message has been pushed that high cholesterol levels spell out inevitable heart disease, and that we should all switch to eating habits that lower them.

Yet how many people know what cholesterol is, and why it should be so apparently dangerous? My guess is very few. Fewer still have been given the unbiased facts about it, and most do not know how to go about lowering their cholesterol levels. This chapter tries to put all this right.

First, it is important to understand that it is *normal* to have cholesterol in the bloodstream. It is a fatty substance used by the body to maintain the integrity of several important organs, such as the liver and brain, and is a 'building brick' in the construction of complex fat-based substances such as cortisone and sex hormones.

So we cannot do without cholesterol completely. We do, however, need to keep its levels in the blood within certain limits. When they are too high, the excess cholesterol appears to be deposited, along with other fats (called lipids) in the walls of the blood vessels, as plaques of atheroma, as explained in Chapter 2. Atheroma leads to heart attacks. So there is a good case for lowering cholesterol levels in people in whom they are too high. The problem, until recently, centred upon the definition of high. However, that has now been settled by such important authorities as the US National Heart Lung and Blood Institute, the Study Group of the European Atherosclerosis Society, and the World Health Organization MONICA Project (*MON*itoring trends *In CA*rdiovascular disease).

Cholesterol levels are measures – from a simple blood test – in millimoles per litre of serum (mmol/l). The experts agree that they are becoming moderately high when they are above 5.2 mmol/l, and need definite attention above 6.5 mmol/l. A person is defined as 'hyperlipidaemic' (with a serious high blood fat level disorder needing medical treatment) if he or she has a cholesterol level above 7.8 mmol/l. The aim for everybody is to keep the cholesterol level between around 4 and 5 mmol/l.

All this advice sounds definite and accurate enough on the surface, but there are practical problems. For a start, if these figures were adhered to, then more than half the population of the United Kingdom, and many other developed countries, would need some form of treatment to lower their cholesterol levels.

All this advice sounds definite and accurate enough on the surface, but there are practical problems. For a start, if these figures were adhered to, then more than half the population of the United Kingdom, and many other developed countries, would need some form of treatment to lower their cholesterol levels.

How do we know if our cholesterol levels are too high? It is not easy. Like high blood pressure, there are no symptoms – until perhaps that fatal heart attack. Some, but not all, hyperlipidaemic patients develop fatty lumps in the skin around the eyes. The only way to be sure is to have the blood test. Everyone over 40 should have one: this is *especially important* for close relatives of people who have had heart attacks in their early and middle adult life.

The Dundee study

In 1989, Dr Hugh Tunstall-Pedoe and colleagues, of Dundee, reported that three-quarters of more than 10,000 men and women aged between 25 and 64 throughout Scotland had cholesterol levels above 5.2 mmol/l. More than a third were over the 6.5 mmol/l mark, and around one in ten was above 7.8 mmol/l. The values rose with age until the 60s in both sexes, levelling off a little earlier in the men.

Scotland, along with Sweden, has the unenviable record of recording the highest death rates from heart attacks in the world, so that these high figures could be said to confirm what the Dundee team already knew – that we Scots are an unhealthy lot! But it was not as simple as that.

Dr Tunstall-Pedoe compared his results with those from other parts of Britain, and found them to be similar. He suggested that they reflected the true position, not just in Scotland, but also elsewhere in Europe and North America.

It would be easy to conclude from these results that there is no need to check cholesterol level before giving advice on lowering it. As cholesterol levels are too high in the vast majority of people then, the argument goes, we may as well save the time and energy that would be used in testing for them, and spread the low cholesterol gospel to *everyone*.

For Dr Tunstall-Pedoe, this is the correct answer. The advice on lowering cholesterol levels, he wrote, can be given safely to everybody. It means advice on better nutrition, encouragement and training – of which more later – and could not do any harm. He suggested that in Britain, a 'national nutrition and lipid-lowering policy be launched'. He condemned the increasing demand for one-off cholesterol measurements as inappropriate.

The Renfrew/Paisley study

Other experts have reservations. At the same time as Dr Tunstall-Pedoe was working in Glasgow and Edinburgh, Dr Christopher Isles and his colleagues were studying the progress of 15,000 men and women in Renfrew and Paisley, to the south-west of Glasgow. Dr Isles' group came to the same conclusion as Dr Tunstall-Pedoe about the link between cholesterol and heart disease. The higher the cholesterol levels, the more deaths there were from heart disease.

However, there was a snag. The people with the lowest cholesterol levels (below 4 mmol/l) tended to have more cancer than the others. Most of the excess deaths were in men with lung cancer, but even when this was corrected for by removing the smokers, there was still a definite link between low cholesterol and cancer rates.

In the Isles study, the lowest overall death rate, including both heart attacks and cancers, was in those with a cholesterol level around 5.6 mmol/l. It would appear, from these figures, that it would be wrong to advise the whole population to reduce their cholesterol levels. For a small number, that advice may well reduce their risk of heart attack, but could also increase other risks.

The answer, according to Dr Isles, must be to concentrate such advice on people only with the highest cholesterol concentrations – say above 6 mmol/l – until more is known about the possible risks of bringing cholesterol levels down too low. Dr Isles agrees that it is difficult to decide what came first in his subjects, the cancer or the low cholesterol. If the cancer caused the low cholesterol (so that the link was the result of his including by chance people who aleady had cancer, as yet undiagnosed, in the study), then lowering cholesterol levels would not do any harm, even when they start out in the low range. It is a different matter if low cholesterol levels can actually initiate a cancerous change in an organ.

How do I stand on this issue? On balance, along with Dr Tunstall-Pedoe. Asking people to change to a sensible system of eating, with the aim of reducing cholesterol levels, will help the vast majority. Most will start with high cholesterol levels, and advice on diet and exercise will only do good by bringing them down into the normal range.

The same advice given to someone whose cholesterol level is already on the low side will hardly alter it further; at this level, eating habits are probably already reasonable and inheritance, rather than nutrition, is likely to be the dominating feature in setting the cholesterol level. It is impossible to alter that!

Cholesterol testing

The Coronary Prevention Group, a group of British doctors set up to try to lower our disastrous heart attack figures, has come to a conclusion somewhere between the two. In 1989, their Chairman, Professor Geoffrey Rose, of the London School of Hygiene and Tropical Medicine, called for the British National Health Service to introduce cholesterol testing in three stages.

The first step was for general practitioners to assess *all* their patients for risk of a coronary attack – on positive family history, smoking, high blood pressure and obesity (more about that in a moment).

Second came cholesterol measurement for those identified at high risk from this first assessment. Patients with high blood cholesterol levels would then be given extra advice, and offered drug treatment (more about this later, too), only if the cholesterol concentrations failed to respond to the appropriate changes in behaviour.

Third, and only after testing those presumed to be at high risk, the tests should be extended to the rest of the population. This should be coupled with advice to everyone, regardless of their cholesterol level, on how to reduce their risk of coronary disease.

The group was concerned that testing for cholesterol alone would be ineffective without the availability of staff with time to spend on giving detailed and effective advice. It would be wrong, they emphasized, for doctors to resort to drug treatment too early, as a substitute for making sure that patients follow the correct lifestyle. 'Treatment through lifestyle change,' they concluded, 'is always preferable to drug treatment, and should always be the first resort.'

Changing the cholesterol risk

Can people lower cholesterol levels just by altering their diet? The answer to that must be a very definite 'yes'. When a simple cholesterol-lowering diet was offered to a group of London civil servants, the proportion of those with cholesterol values below 5.2 mmol/l rose from only 5 per cent to 29 per cent. So it can be done. Those who try it find, very often, that they actually enjoy the new eating style, and the way they feel on it.

Cholesterol reaches the bloodstream from two sources: in the food we eat (as in eggs) or from our own livers, where it is made from fats (mainly animal fats) taken in food. Dietary cholesterol is probably much less important than eating animal fats in producing atheroma, so that, except in people with very high cholesterol levels, high cholesterol foods such as eggs and animal liver need not be too restricted. Nevertheless, two or three eggs a week, and liver no more than once a week are probably enough for any adult.

What really matters, however, is how much fat we eat. We get our fats from red meat and dairy products, such as cream, cheese, butter and full cream milk. The authorities now recommend that dietary fats should only account for between 30 and 35 per cent of the total calorie intake – this is far lower than most British diets.

This is especially true for children. For most British children 40 per cent of their food energy supply, measured as calories, is taken in as fat: this figure rises to 50 per cent or more for junk food addicts. This is potentially tragic, because atheroma starts in childhood, and all those hamburgers and chips are likely to lead to heart trouble in relatively early adulthood.

For parents worried about themselves and their children, there are immediate steps to be taken. The first is to grill, rather than fry, foods. Very small children, say up to the age of five, may need full cream milk as a source of energy. After then, however, it is better for everyone to drink or cook with semi-skimmed or skimmed, rather than whole milk.

For the most part, butter and hard margarines should be largely replaced by low fat soft spreads made from buttermilk and skimmed milk, or by soft margarines made from polyunsaturated vegetable oils. If you must eat cheese, choose cottage-type makes with low fat content, rather than traditional cheddar.

Vegetable oils, rather than lard or butter, should be used for cooking; and fish, poultry and vegetables should replace, as far as possible, meats and dairy products. There is no need to cut out beef, lamb and pork altogether, but it is wise to eat them on a maximum of two days a week, and to cut off all the obvious fat before eating them.

Here a point should be made about osteoporosis. This has been suggested as the 'down side' of low fat food. The loss of bone mineral after the menopause, which leads to hip fracture and bowed spines in older women, has been blamed on diets deficient in calcium and fats. This is not true. The progress of osteoporosis is relentless regardless of diet. Women who wish to keep their bones strong and well mineralized could not do better than to keep active (exercise is the best way to keep bones strong) and to have a diet full of good quality vegetables – just the diet that will also protect their hearts.

In fact, the ideal diet is to go Italian. Italian food is not only among the best in the world, it is certainly the healthiest! Italians cook mainly in olive oil, eat plenty of high quality vegetables and fruit, their fish is superb, and they eat meat sparingly. Their vegetable soups are not only tasty, they are virtually fat-free and filling, too. One advantage of eating them as a starter is that you will eat less in your main course.

Their pastas are starchy, rather than sugary, and that is all to the good. Even the garlic helps; garlic and to a lesser extent, onions, contain substances that tend to prevent clotting. Eating garlic every day may not make you popular with your closest friends (unless they are eating it, too), but it could help you live longer!

The most important thing about this change is that it is a *positive* one, towards expanding food experiences. It is not a question of cutting down on food. You will find that you will eat just as much, and be just as satisfied, after a high vegetable, high fruit, fish or poultry meal with pasta, or say, a baked potato, than after the meat and two veg and pudding and custard so beloved of the British.

And the new tastes you will encounter on the way will be a revelation. Experiment with spices and throw away the salt cellar, and you will soon find your enjoyment of, and enthusiasm for, food enhanced – without putting on weight.

Of course, not everyone can or wants to eat Italian-style. There are British alternatives – such as that baked potato instead of pasta, and onions instead of garlic. There are alternatives that will serve just as well. Again, make fish or poultry your main source of protein. Grill them, or shallow fry them in oil: for a bit of extra taste, try frying them in oatmeal. Don't reuse the oil more than three times: repeated use turns oils from 'unsaturated' to 'saturated'.

The last ten years have seen a revolution in the vegetables and fruits that are available in British shops. We are no longer limited to cabbage, sprouts, carrots and peas, or apples, plums and pears. Vegetables are no longer seasonal. We can buy cauliflower, broccoli, courgettes, peppers, aubergines, avocados (full of fat, perhaps, but of the right sort), and a myriad of other vegetables all the year round.

The same goes for fruits: think of the variety of oranges now on the shelves, and the abundance of pineapples, grapes, melons and kiwi fruits. We can even enjoy fresh pawpaws, mangoes or guavas.

So changing your style of eating (abolish the thought that it is a 'diet') to include all these new possibilities should be looked on as an adventure, rather than an imposition – as a positive step to a much more enjoyable life.

Misconceptions about obesity

Before turning to the next chapter, some common misconceptions about food and eating should be put to rest. The first has to be about obesity. Fat people are more likely to have a heart attack than thin people – but the relationship is not a straightforward one. And many thin people still have heart attacks. Eating too much, and exercising too little, causes obesity and coronary disease, but you can still have coronary disease if you are thin by eating the wrong things.

What does this prove? It is better to be of normal weight than to be overweight, but obesity of itself may not be a direct cause of coronary disease. The fact is that if you are overweight, your blood levels of cholesterol are usually higher than normal, and it is this, and not simply being too fat, that makes a heart attack more likely.

The consequence of this is that just reducing weight alone, without also reducing your cholesterol levels, may not help. Of course, losing excess weight will always make you feel and look better, and you will be happier with your own body image. It will also probably reduce your chance of stroke and reduce any high blood pressure you may have – but unless you also reduce your blood cholesterol level, your chances of avoiding a heart attack will not increase.

Here is a typical 45-year-old British male factory worker as an example. Three years ago he was developing middle-aged spread. At around 3 stone (20 kg) overweight, he felt he had to do something about his health – so he bought a dog, and started taking it out for a walk every night. The extra exercise, he reasoned, would take off the weight, and he could carry on with his eating habits of a lifetime.

He was right. He started to enjoy the exercise and added to it by joining his wife, twice a week, at the local swimming pool. Now he was just the right weight for his height of 5 feet 10 inches (1.7 m) – just under 12 stones (126 kg).

Yet when he came for his 'well man' visit, his doctor was very concerned. His cholesterol level was 7.1 mmol/l, which put him in the top quarter for heart attack risk. That, along with his ten-a-day cigarette consumption, and a slightly raised blood pressure, gave him a one in three chance of a heart attack in the next five years.

Needless to say, he did not think much of these odds! Asked about his eating habits, he confessed to a 'good fry-up' for breakfast most mornings, cheese or bacon sandwiches for lunch, tea and chocolate biscuits in the afternoon break, and a typical dinner of 'meat and two veg' followed by pudding or tart and custard every evening. He might finish the day with a toasted cheese snack and a milk chocolate drink.

He rarely ate fish, his vegetables were confined to a few cooked 'greens', and he never bothered with fruit. Potatoes were usually eaten as chips, or mashed with cream and butter – a special favourite.

It took some persuading for him and his wife to change the habits of a lifetime – but it worked. His mornings now start with cereal, such as muesli, or porridge, taken with skimmed milk or yoghurt, plus toasted wholemeal bread, spread with jam or marmalade. His lunchtime sandwiches are now filled with chicken, turkey, sardines or mackerel paté, which he follows with an apple or pear or an orange. This now does him until the evening, except for his afternoon cup of tea (he has abandoned his chocolate biscuit).

His dinner is now much more varied than before, ranging from pastas to grills, stews and even curries, so that his chips and mash have been replaced by rice and pasta or potatoes baked or boiled in their jackets. At least three times a week his main course is a fish – preferably an 'oily' one, such as herring, mackerel, sardines, trout and salmon. Now that salmon prices have slumped below cod prices, he and his wife do not see it as a luxury item. He eats so well that he doesn't find it necessary to take anything just before bedtime, except, perhaps, a cup of tea and some fruit. His weight is steady, but he does not feel he has been put on a diet, or is eating too little.

The effect on his cholesterol has been dramatic. In three months it fell down to around 5 mmol/l – well within the normal range. He has also stopped smoking. His blood pressure has also swung down into the normal range, possibly because his salt consumption has fallen along with his fat consumption. He feels fitter, too, with more zest for life. It is only now that he feels so much better that he realizes how unfit he still was, even after losing the weight.

This combination of the lower cholesterol, the non-smoking, and the lowered blood pressure has greatly improved his chance of survival. Now the statistics say that he has less than one chance in fifteen of having a heart attack in the next five years. That is a five-fold reduction in risk, about which he, his wife and his doctor are all very happy!

This story could be told a million times or more around Britain and other developed countries, with very little variation. It is never too late for anyone to change – it just means a little initial effort in taking the decision. Once people take the plunge, and start to try all the new ways they can eat, then few return to the old habits. The first step is always the hardest.

Drugs to lower cholesterol

Of course, not everyone has the discipline to change a lifestyle so completely that they can lower their cholesterol levels as far as they need. And for some people, born with the tendency to a high blood cholesterol, it remains high even if they adhere very strictly to a low-fat lifestyle. For them the only answer is to take cholesterol-lowering drugs.

Trials reported in the mid-1990s all showed that the newest of this class of drugs, the 'statins', both reduce cholesterol levels and consistently prevent heart attacks and strokes – lowering their rates by around a third. The authorities on cholesterol, the British Hyperlipidaemia Association (BHA) and the European Atherosclerosis Society (EAS), have come to a consensus on what doctors should do about patients with high cholesterol levels.

The desirable total cholesterol (TC) level is no more than 5.2 mmol/l of blood. Within this figure the 'low density lipoprotein cholesterol' (LDL) level should be no more than 3.5 mmol/l if the person possesses other risk factors for heart disease such as high blood pressure or smokes. The BHA and EAC counsel doctors to treat people with TC levels between 5.2 and 6.5 mmol/l with weight reduction, a diet low in saturated fat and cholesterol, and high in fibre. Those with TC levels between 6.5 and 7.8 mmol/l should have a rigorous trial of diet, but be switched to drugs if they do not respond with a steep drop in TC. People with TCs above 7.8 mmol/l should be treated with both diet and drugs. These people may need two drugs of different types to lower their cholesterol levels satisfactorily.

According to the trial results, the most effective group of cholesterol-lowering drugs is the 'statins'. They include atorvastatin, cerivastatin, fluvastatin, pravastatin and simvastatin. They are not all exactly alike: they have different doses and different side-effects, so that one statin may suit one person better than another. The commonest side-effect is muscle pain, although this seems to be less severe with the newer drugs, such as atorvastatin. A complete list of cholesterol-lowering drugs is given in Appendix 2.

As anyone reading this far will already have realized, however, cholesterol alone is only part of the story. It cannot be taken in isolation from smoking, exercise and blood pressure – and alcohol consumption has also to be considered. The next three chapters take them in order, and offer practical advice on how you can change them for the better.

41

4
Smoking and drinking

This chapter pulls no punches. Smoking is a stupid, suicidal habit with absolutely nothing to commend it. It not only puts you at high risk of a heart attack, it gives you chronic bronchitis and emphysema, and increases your chances of cancers of the lung, the kidney, and bladder. It can destroy the delicate blood vessels in your legs, so that you can be left with gangrene and amputations, and it will raise your blood pressure, making you more susceptible to strokes.

It gives people a sallow, unhealthy look, and wrinkles. By the time they are 40, women smokers look ten years older than their non-smoking sisters. By 60, many of them are already dead. Cancer of the lung and heart attacks, both of them directly due to their smoking habit, cause far more early deaths in women than anything else.

Virtually all adult smokers started the habit as teenagers, when they were far too immature to think about the long-term consequences. If you are a non-smoker at 20 it is odds on that you will remain so for the rest of your life; by this time most people have learned sense.

The first cigarette makes you nauseated, dizzy and ill, as the poisons in the smoke enter the brain. New smokers have to be persuaded to continue by their tobacco-addicted colleagues – one of the signs of true addicts is that they want to 'switch on' their friends. Within days, the drug addiction takes hold. Now they feel unwell when they do not have a smoke, because the withdrawal symptoms take over. From then on, it is downhill all the way. No matter how strong the smoker's will, after a few years, he or she will be smoking between 20 and 60 a day.

Just imagine if cigarettes were new: that someone were now to come to the market for the first time with a product with such effects! No food or drugs authority in the world would entertain them. They might even be prosecuted for deliberately trying to damage the nation's health.

Sadly, tobacco has been with us for a long time. Its bad effects have been recognized for nearly as long. Here is King James VI of

Scotland (James I of England) sounding off about it in the early seventeenth century:

> Loathsome to the eye, hateful to the nose, harmful to the brain, dangerous to the lungs, and in the black stinking fume thereof nearest resembling the horrible Stygian smoke of the pit that is bottomless.

To a doctor like myself, who has had to comfort so many families in which smoking has directly led to the deaths of men and women in their 40s and 50s, it is frankly incredible that anyone should wish to light up a single cigarette. The very fact that smoking has been so much more important than life itself for people is unbelievable – yet around 40 per cent of the population still smoke.

How, exactly, does smoking harm the heart? Tobacco smoke contains carbon monoxide and nicotine. The first is a gas that poisons the red blood cells, so that they cannot deliver the oxygen the heart needs. It also poisons the heart muscle, so that it cannot beat properly. It is the gas that used to kill people in ovens fuelled by coal gas, and is the gas which still kills suicides who use car exhausts.

Nicotine stimulates the body to make adrenaline, which makes the heart beat faster: this puts extra strain on it, especially if it is already affected by carbon monoxide. It also causes the coronary arteries to narrow, so that the blood flow through them slows down. It raises the blood sugar and blood fat levels, thickening the blood and promoting atheroma.

Both nicotine and carbon monoxide encourage the blood to clot, which multiplies the risk even more. Not only that, there is good evidence that years of smoking directly damage the walls of the small blood vessels, and accelerates the progress of atheroma. Carbon monoxide-affected red blood cells are also stiffened, so that they cannot pass smoothly through the smallest blood vessels.

Add to that the tars that smoking deposits in the lungs, which further reduce the ability of red blood cells to carry the vital oxygen, and the scars in the lungs that make it more difficult to breathe, and you have a multiple formula for disaster.

If you are not yet convinced, then consider the following facts:

- Smoking causes more deaths from heart attacks than it does deaths from any other disease, including chronic bronchitis and lung cancer.

- People who smoke cigarettes have a two or three times greater risk of a fatal heart attack than non-smokers. The risk rises in parallel with the numbers of cigarettes smoked.
- Men under the age of 45 who smoke 25 or more cigarettes a day have a ten to fifteen times greater chance of death from heart attack than non-smokers.
- In the developed countries, such as Britain, one-third of men die before they reach 65, most from smoking-related diseases. That means one-third of all married women are widows before they can enjoy retirement with their husbands.
- About 40 per cent of all heavy smokers die before they reach 65. Of the 60 per cent still alive then, many are disabled by bronchitis, angina, heart failure, or because of leg amputations – all because of their smoking habit. Only 10 per cent survive in reasonable health to the age of 75. Most non-smokers reach 75 in good health.
- Smoking takes a terrible toll in other ways than heart attacks. In Britain, 40 per cent of all cancer deaths in men are due to lung cancer. It is very rare in non-smokers: of 441 British male doctors who died of lung cancer, only seven had never smoked. Only one non-smoker in 60 develops lung cancer: the figure for heavy smokers is one in six!
- Other cancers more common in smokers than in non-smokers include tumours of the tongue, throat, larynx, pancreas, kidney, bladder and cervix. About one-third of all cancers are caused directly by smoking.

Now that you have read this far, you may be thinking of giving up the weed. If you are, then strengthen your resolve – don't weaken it with the host of excuses that doctors hear all the time from their patients. Here are a sample – there are plenty more, all of them spurious:

- *My uncle/father/grandfather smoked 20 a day and lived until he was 75.*

Everyone knows someone like that. But they forget all the others they also knew, who died long before their time. The chances are that you will be one of them, rather than one of the very few lucky ones.

- *People who don't smoke also have heart attacks.*

True: there are other causes of heart attacks, but it remains a fact that 70 per cent of all people under 65 years old admitted to coronary care units with heart attacks are smokers, as are 91 per cent of patients considered for coronary artery bypass surgery for angina.

- *Moderation in everything is no bad thing, and I only smoke moderately.*

That is just nonsense. Do people accept moderation in lead poisoning, dangerous driving, radiation or exposure to asbestos (which causes very many fewer deaths than smoking)? Of course not. Younger men who are only moderate smokers have a much higher risk of heart attack than non-smokers of the same age. There is no lower, safe limit to cigarette smoking.

- *I can cut down, rather than stop.*

You may be able to, but it won't do much good. People who cut down on the number of cigarettes usually take more inhalations from each cigarette, leave a smaller butt, and end up with the same amount of carbon monoxide and nicotine in their bloodstream. The only answer is to stop.

- *I am just as likely to be run over crossing the road as dying from smoking.*

In Britain about fifteen people die on the roads every day. This compares with a daily toll of 100 people from lung cancer, 100 from chronic bronchitis, and 100 from heart attacks – almost all of which are due to smoking. Of every 1000 young men who smoke, on average one will be murdered, six will die on the roads, and 250 will die before their time because of their smoking.

- *I have to die of something.*

In my experience this is always said by someone in good health. It is rare for anyone to say it once he or she has developed angina or had a heart attack. And they change their tune very quickly if they start coughing up blood!

- *I don't want to live to be old, anyway.*

Our definition of 'old' seems to change as we grow older! Most of us would like to live a long time, but none of us wants to be old. And if we take care of ourselves on the way to becoming old, we have at least laid the groundwork for a good chance of enjoying our old age.

• *I'd rather die of a heart attack than something else.*

Most of us would like to die in a 'clean' way. That is all very fine, but many heart attack victims leave a grieving partner in their early 50s to face 20 or 30 years of loneliness. Is that really what you wish?

• *Stress, not smoking, is the main cause of heart attacks.*

Who has the most stress? The top executive or the single parent on a low income struggling to make ends meet? Stress is not only difficult to measure, it is very difficult to relate to heart attack rates in any meaningful way. In any case, the stress is there, to be coped with somehow: smoking is an extra burden on your heart that can never help.

Dr Barrie Smith, a consultant chest physician from Sandwell in the English West Midlands, has pointed out that the Prime Minister's job must be one of the most stressful in Britain. Only one British Prime Minister in the last 100 years has died under the age of 70. To quote Dr Smith: '*It is not burning the candle at both ends that causes harm, rather it is burning the cigarette at one end.*'

• *I'll stop when I start to develop heart disease.*

That would be fine, if the first sign of heart disease for many people were not a full-blown heart attack from which 40 per cent die in the first four hours! It's too late to think of stopping smoking then!

• *I'll put on weight if I give up smoking.*

You probably will, because your appetite will return and you will be able to taste food again. So take the opportunity to make that change in your diet you promised yourself after reading the last chapter – your new-found enjoyment in food will help you do it. If you do put on weight, it will probably only be temporary, and in any case, the health risks of gaining weight are much lower than those of continuing to smoke.

• *I enjoy smoking, and don't want to give it up.*

Is that really true? Are you sure that this is not just an excuse, because it sounds better than admitting that you can't stop? Ask yourself what the real pleasure is in smoking, and see if you can be honest with yourself.

- *Cigarettes settle my nerves. If I stopped I would have to take Valium.*

Smoking is certainly a prop, something like a baby's dummy. The ritual of the packet, the lighter, the fondling of the cigarette, holding it in the mouth, the need to do something with the hands or to fend off boredom or loneliness; these are all reasons for smoking. However, it solves nothing. It does not remove the cause of any stress, and can only make things worse in the long term because of its proven bad effect on health.

As the smoking habit continues, the mechanics of the habit take up more of your time, affecting efficiency, vitality and enjoyment of other pleasures. Non-smoking friends are more likely nowadays to object, and that increases, rather than reduces, anxiety. This is probably building up, anyway, as you become more worried about your health. That morning cough which always develops is an early sign of chronic bronchitis. From then on, no one can say that smoking relieves anxiety – with each cigarette you are reminding yourself of the damage you may be doing.

Interestingly, the anxiety-prone person who worries about his or her smoking has a good chance of giving up.

- *I'll change to a pipe or cigars – they are safer.*

It is true that lifelong pipe and cigar smokers are at very little increased risk of heart attack, but they still have five times more lung cancer and ten times more chronic bronchitis than non-smokers. Unfortunately, cigarette smokers who switch to pipes or cigars continue to be at high risk of a heart attack, probably because they continue to inhale.

- *I've been smoking now for 30 years – it is too late to give up.*

It certainly is *not* too late, at whatever age you stop. The risk of sudden death from a heart attack if you have no history of heart disease drops steeply, until after a year or two it is the same as if you were always a non-smoker. If you smoke until your first heart attack and survive, then stop, that will reduce your chance of a second attack. If you carry on smoking, then make sure that your life insurance is in order! Stopping smoking also reduces the risk of lung cancer, but it takes much longer to have an effect: after fifteen years it falls by 80 per cent.

- *I wish I could stop – I've tried everything, but nothing has worked.*

Stopping smoking is not easy, unless you really want to do it. That means putting some effort into it yourself, rather than thinking someone else can do it for you. That, in turn, means you have to be motivated. If the last few pages have not motivated you, then I do not know what will!

Stopping smoking

So you have decided you must stop smoking, or you want to help your partner to stop. How do you go about it?

Most important of all is to find the right reason to stop. No one ever stops who does not want to stop. Many who would like to stop fail because they are not fully convinced of the need. So the first task is to find the motivation that will make the smoker – yourself or your partner – stick to the resolve.

Motivation differs from person to person and from age to age. For example, young people care little for the health risks. They may even be attracted to the risk, as a dangerous, exciting aspect of smoking. Middle age and sickness are too remote: they don't make the link with themselves.

Instead, for teenagers and young adults, the best attack on smoking is the way it makes them look and smell. Smoking is dirty, and leaves a stale smell on the breath, clothes and hair. It is also environmentally polluting, and exploits Third World poverty to the benefit of big multinational businesses – very much a concern of today's younger generation. Which teenager likes the feeling that he or she is being 'ripped off' by one of the big multinationals?

What does the young environmentally conscious smoker think when he or she hears that Third World land which could be used for food is instead used for tobacco – and that the profits go into arms, liquor and luxury electrical goods for the few, instead of food or agricultural machines? This happens in regimes of the left or the right. Pakistan uses 120,000 acres, and Brazil uses half a million acres, of the most fertile land to grow tobacco to satisfy the needs of the developed world.

Not only that, the tobacco companies are vigorously promoting their wares to Third World populations, adding smoking-regulated diseases to their burden of malnutrition and poor social conditions. Faced with these facts, no youngster who smokes can claim to be concerned about the health of the Third World. That is often as persuasive an argument as any on health or looks.

For many older women, appearance can be the key to stopping. Smoking ages people prematurely. This is not just expressed in more wrinkles, but in the whole complexion. Smoking shuts down the skin blood vessels, so that the face loses its healthy pink colour, turning to white or grey. Smoking women who buy expensive facial creams and beauty treatments could save themselves the money by stopping smoking.

Such rapid ageing extends to the hormonal balance in women, too. Women smokers undergo an earlier menopause; it may even start in the mid-30s. This can destroy the plans of the businesswoman who decides to postpone her family for a while. That 'while' can be an eternity.

For adult men, the primary motivation to stop must be health. The statistics on survival beyond 60 for the regular male smoker are simply frightening. Around a third of men do not live to enjoy the money they have saved all their lives through their pensions. If that doesn't convince them, they should think of their wives, who will live alone for the last 20 or more years of their lives. There are few merry widows outside operettas.

Once you have the motivation, how do you go about stopping? First of all, make sure that your aim is to stop, and not just to cut down. Then decide whether you wish to stop all at once, or plan a gradual retreat. Both systems will work, provided you are convinced enough.

Many smokers find, to their surprise, that stopping suddenly is very easy. They take all the cigarettes in their possession and in the house, scrunch them up, and throw them in the bin. Then they resolve never to buy any more, and always say 'no', without thinking about it, to whoever offers them a cigarette.

General de Gaulle went further: he announced to the whole French nation, on television, that he had stopped smoking. After that, he would never dare light up, in case a member of the Press caught him at it and exposed him as a fraud or backslider! Most people could do something similar, in front of friends; in today's relatively anti-smoking climate, that would evoke sympathy and support, rather than sneers or sniggers.

Of course, stopping all of a sudden raises the bogey of withdrawal symptoms. They can vary from the severe – with agitation, irritation, nervousness and sleeplessness – to nothing at all. People who have to give up smoking for medical reasons, such as admission to a coronary care unit, hardly ever have withdrawal symptoms which suggest that they are psychological, rather than physical. In any case, the desire to smoke usually subsides after a week or two, as the feeling of well-being induced by the dropping blood levels of carbon monoxide, nicotine and tarry chemicals takes over.

However, if you just cannot do it all in one go, then plan to stop gradually. The way to do that is to write it down and stick to it. Make a 'stop' day, two or three weeks ahead, preferably during a long weekend or holiday. Be aware of every cigarette smoked, and give it a value, from one to ten, about its importance to you. That will show you how important it is to smoke at that time of day.

Keep your cigarettes in a drawer, or on a shelf, not on your person, or in your handbag. That will make it an extra effort to go and light one. Start your planned withdrawal by cutting out your 'best' cigarette of the day – such as the first one on rising in the morning, or the one with the coffee break. Then delay the first cigarette of the day by one hour each day.

Carry chewing gum or low calorie 'nibbles', such as pieces of carrot or celery, to chew when you feel the need for a smoke. Get a friend to support and encourage you, and monitor your progress each day; use a graph, if you like, to monitor the dropping number of cigarettes.

If you find that you still can't stop, then don't despair. Many people have to try several times before they finally succeed. They usually find that it gets easier with each effort, until they finally break the habit altogether. You can always ask your family doctor for help. Since 2000, aids for stopping smoking have diversified from nicotine chewing gums to sprays, patches and Zyban, a prescription drug that interferes with the function of that part of the brain thought to be involved in maintaining nicotine addiction. They are all useful in helping to stave off withdrawal symptoms, but they are no substitute for your own determination to succeed. If you do use aids to stop smoking, you must realize that it depends on you, not the aid, or on anyone trying to help you. That goes for chewing gum, acupuncture and hypnosis – none of them have any magical properties. They only serve to support your own determination: they cannot bolster a weak will.

Realize, too, that stopping is not a single end in itself. Smoking has been part of your life, probably for years. You feel it has relaxed or stimulated you. You will have to replace it with a new, positive, attitude to life. Take plenty of exercise during the critical period: that will help to relieve the tension and stop you putting on weight. Take plenty of fluids, such as fruit juices, and eat more fruit: you will find the new taste exciting and stimulating. Try a new hobby, with new friends. And take special care not to succumb to temptation at the time of what was your 'best' cigarette.

From the time you reach your planned 'stop' day, the break must be complete. You will never buy or accept another cigarette. Never risk 'just one', even at smoky parties where the alcohol flows freely, and your resistance is low. Be especially on your guard on these occasions. If you accept one cigarette, you will be back where you started within weeks.

You owe making the effort to stop smoking to your heart and your future – and to the future of your family or partner. You will not be on your own. Around a million Britons have given up the habit in each of the last ten or so years. Only one in three adults now smokes. When you stop, you will simply be joining the sensible majority.

Alcohol

It is plain from the last few pages that there is no such thing as moderate smoking. Every cigarette has the potential to do the heart harm. Is the same true of alcohol?

That is very difficult to answer. First, it has to be conceded that there is no evidence to link moderate amounts of alcohol with heart disease. Alcohol tends to open up arteries, rather than close them, so some doctors have even argued that a little alcohol may do 'heart' patients good.

However, it all depends on what is meant by a 'little', and on whether the drinker can stick to the rules. A little can so easily become a lot!

Probably the group of doctors to have done most to investigate the effects and ill-effects of measured amounts of alcohol are the team led by Professor Roger Williams, of the Liver Unit at London's King's College Hospital. Over many years they have studied the drinking habits of thousands of people, and they have finally come to definite conclusions, which are now used as standards for the guidance of doctors all over the world.

Classically, doctors have been taught that the main organs attacked by alcohol are the liver and the brain. Too much alcohol causes cirrhosis and even cancer of the liver, and can damage the brain cells, leading to loss of intellect and even insanity.

So how much is too much? The King's College team have defined that very clearly. They talk of standard 'units' of alcohol. One unit is equivalent to a half pint (500 ml) of beer or lager, one glass of wine, one measure of fortified wines such as sherry or martini, and a single measure of spirit such as whisky or gin (a half measure in Scotland).

Men, according to the experts, can cope with up to 21 standard units of drink a week. For women the upper weekly limit is only 14 units. (The difference is not just due to their difference in size: it also arises from the need for the liver in women to cope with their sex hormones as well as the alcohol.)

This means that the regular male drinker should take no more than three drinks, and his female counterpart no more than two drinks, on any night. However, even this may be too much, if the drinking goes on every night. Professor Williams' team advise that the body should be given a rest from alcohol on at least three days a week.

This advice was originally given to help people avoid liver and brain damage, but it is now becoming clear that it holds good for the heart, too.

There is nothing to suggest that alcohol in excess helps to cause heart attacks, in the sense that it might narrow the coronary arteries, accelerate atheroma or make the blood more viscous. It does not increase the blood's tendency to clot. It may even open up blood vessels a little – this is the cause of an alcoholic flush. So, superficially, alcohol could be said to help, rather than promote heart attacks. This, in fact, used to be the advice given by some doctors. They suggested to patients who already had heart disease that 'a little drink every now and then' might do good.

Unfortunately that advice is wrong! The proof of that was given by Dr Gareth Beevers, of Dudley Road Hospital, Birmingham. Dr Beevers is an internationally known specialist in hypertension (high blood pressure). A review of thousands of patients with hypertension established a very strong link between alcohol consumption and high blood pressure: the more people drank, the higher the pressure.

This surprised many doctors, who felt that alcohol might if anything lower the pressure. Dr Beevers proved, however, that alcohol had a special, direct effect on the heart, even when taken in moderate doses. Many moderate drinkers had enlarged hearts, high blood pressure and a poor heart reserve in times of crisis.

The conclusion had to be that if you are a drinker, and have a heart problem, such as angina or a full blown heart attack, then the alcohol will always make that worse, rather than better. For the person with angina it is probably better to be teetotal than to take alcohol as a 'stimulant'. In fact, Dr Beevers' work suggested that alcohol may appear to the drinker to be a stimulant, but it is in fact a depressant.

So how much can one drink without causing harm? For people who are healthy, and obey all the rules, such as not smoking, exercising well, eating correctly, and who do not have high blood pressure or diabetes, then the King's College figures apply. They can drink up to two or three units per day, perhaps four times a week.

For the person with high blood pressure or angina, or who has had a previous heart attack, then this may be too much. Where alcohol is concerned, each case should be taken on its merits. My advice is, if you are in one of these categories, that you should talk over your drinking habits very carefully, and honestly, with your specialist.

Looking back on Dr Beevers' work from the vantage point of the year 2000, it seems that opinions on alcohol vary from time to time, but the underlying message remains the same. Today's accepted opinion is that people who drink a little are a little less likely to have heart attacks and strokes than those who drink no alcohol at all. And they are a lot less likely to have them than people who drink more than the standard three drinks a day for men and two drinks a day for women. However, this book is meant for people who already have heart problems: these risk statistics refer to people in normal health. Interestingly they come from population studies in Bordeaux (home of red wine), Munich (home of beer) and Edinburgh (home of whisky). There is no evidence that alcohol is beneficial to people whose hearts are already at risk, and it may be harmful. So the advice remains, drink only in moderation.

A last word about alcohol. Probably the busiest days of the year for family doctors are those immediately after a national feast day or holiday. I'm thinking of Christmas in England, or New Year's Day in Scotland – or of special occasions, like a reunion or anniversary party. It is at times like these that people overeat – usually a meal full of animal fats – and over drink as well. The inhibitions are down, everyone is merry, and they go to bed full of food and drink.

During the night, all the conditions for shutting off a blood vessel in the brain or the heart are fulfilled – the fat in the bloodstream makes the blood flow more sluggish, the blood's tendency to clot will rise, the strain on that little plaque of atheroma will be that little bit greater, and the alcohol will have raised the blood pressure that little bit further. The result, in susceptible people, is the heart attack or stroke in the small morning hours.

I hate to be a killjoy, but if you have taken the trouble to change your lifestyle to protect your heart, it is a great pity to throw it away just because of one night of overindulgence. You can enjoy a party without overeating and drinking too much, and think of how much better you will feel in the morning!

5
Exercise

One of the best books to appear in the 1970s was *The Complete Book of Running* by James Fixx. Fixx was probably the man most responsible for the rise to popularity of running, or jogging. Fixx found himself, in his mid-thirties, with a heart problem, weighing nearly 16 stones (100 kg) and breathless after trying to run 50 metres.

He decided to take up running, and by the time he wrote his book, ten years later, in 1978, he had lost 4 stone (25 kg) in weight, had run the equivalent of once around the Equator, had competed in marathons all around the world, and was running 10 miles (16 km) every day.

By 1984, his book was recommended reading for all people keen to help their general health, and particularly their hearts. That changed overnight when Fixx died, while running, from a heart attack in his late 50s. Exercise is fine and fun, but it should be tempered by the realization that it is not everything, and that there are times when you need to seek other help.

The problem with James was that he believed that he could 'run through' his heart trouble. He became so engrossed in his running schedule that he did not seek help for his increasing angina problems. He had, in fact, severe atheroma, probably a hangover from his overweight days, and maybe complicated by the fact that his father had died, in his 30s, from coronary heart disease. This sort of history suggests that the Fixx family may have inherited a tendency to very high blood fat levels. Nowhere in his book does he mention his own blood cholesterol or fat levels.

Perhaps if he had slowed down a little, and asked for medical advice, he could still be alive today. There are plenty of effective ways to lower cholesterol and to treat angina now, which might have helped prevent that final attack. They will be described in Chapter 6.

It still could be argued that James Fixx was a success story. After all, his exercise allowed him around 20 years of extra life before his heart disease eventually killed him. But the suspicion is still there, that if only he had not been quite so obsessional, he could have lived longer.

So what is the place of exercise if you wish to avoid heart disease, or already have it and do not want to end up like Mr Fixx? For a start, the news is all good. Exercise *is* good for you, even when your heart has been badly affected by previous attacks.

This will surprise many older people who can remember heart victims being asked to rest most of the day, for weeks and months at a stretch. When I qualified in medicine, in 1962, there was a strict routine for all victims of heart attacks. They were kept lying almost flat in bed for between six and twelve weeks.

The idea was that if you 'rested' the heart until the scar of the heart attack healed, the eventual scar would be stronger and smaller, and the eventual recovery would be better. However, the heart attack patient from then on was expected to lead a fairly quiet life.

Perhaps this advice to rest was really a hangover from the Victorian age, when it was fashionable to take to one's bed at the onset of any illness, and to stay there, no matter what, until one was fully 'convalesced'. From the mid-nineteenth century until the 1960s, 'convalescent homes' and 'rest homes' were places where people could relax and laze until they were better from whatever acute illness they were thought to have.

You did not have to be ill to take to your bed. Florence Nightingale and Charles Darwin were two noted Victorians who spent most of their adult lives languishing in bed, suffering from 'neurasthenia', or 'nervous exhaustion'. Such examples made the 'cardiac cripple' almost fashionable. People who had any sort of heart disease were told that they were 'delicate' and must not overexert themselves. Once you had had a heart attack, all sorts of activity were forbidden, including walking upstairs, running or even lovemaking.

All this advice was given on the basis of no facts at all! Because some eminent physicians theorized that rest was good, it was accepted as good. We know different now. We know that the way to strengthen an organ is to use it, not to rest it.

The proof of that is simple. Think of the last time you were ill enough to be forced to stay in bed, say with influenza. After only a few days in bed, how did you feel on the first day up? Weak, shaky, and surprisingly lacking in energy? That was not the aftermath of the virus infection, but the effect of prolonged rest on your leg and back muscles.

When muscles are not used for more than a day or two, they

quickly begin to waste: they lose their stores of energy. The change is only temporary, and they quickly build up their strength again once activity is resumed. However, the longer you rest, the weaker the muscles are, the longer they take to recover, and the more you wish to rest. That starts a vicious circle that can be difficult to break.

The heart is no different from any other muscle in this respect. It needs to be stimulated to keep strong. Working at resting pace all the time will make it difficult for it to step up a gear when it is needed.

Today, therefore, the aim is to keep people with heart trouble as active as their condition will allow. They are asked to exercise on 'treadmills' (really just moving pavement machines used as standard clinic tests) to determine their capabilities. Even if your heart is failing, there is always something you can do to make life more active, and to improve the efficiency of your circulation.

What is true of those who already have heart disease is even more true for the population at large. We human beings developed as hunter-gatherers. We were built to walk for miles, day after day, looking for food. If we sit, inert, for most of the day, we become unfit. Unless, of course, we make sure that we set time aside for exercise. The only argument is about how much exercise we need to keep fit, without going overboard about it, like the late James Fixx.

How fit is your heart?

First of all, you will want to know how fit your heart is. One of the simplest ways to do this is to use the 'Harvard Step Test' where you step up and down on a bench for a few minutes, then see how your heart recovers from the effort.

You can perform this test at home. All you need is a bench 20 inches (50 cm) high or a flight of stairs, and a watch with a second hand. Step from the floor on to the bench or the second step of the stairs (missing out the first) and down again, 30 times a minute for four minutes. Time yourself with the watch, or, if you have one, use a metronome. You must straighten your knee fully at each step up.

If you get too exhausted to carry on, note down the time that you stopped: it will make a difference to your eventual score. The test is quite strenuous, so be cautious. If you experience any problems, such as tightness in the chest, breathing difficulties or chest pain, then *stop immediately*.

As soon as you have finished, sit quietly and take your pulse for a full 30 seconds, starting exactly one minute after you finish. Write down the number of beats immediately, then repeat the 30-second pulse count and writing twice more, starting two minutes after you stopped the exercise, and then again a minute later.

You will find your pulse easiest just above the wrist on the thumb side of the inside of the forearm, between the first tendon and the bone. Use your index and middle fingers to time it.

You can then calculate your 'recovery index'. This is the duration of the exercise in seconds multiplied by 100 divided by double the sum of the three pulse counts.

Take these two examples. Mr A stopped the exercise after three minutes 40 seconds (220 seconds), and his respective pulse rates were 76, 64 and 60. This gives a score of 22,000 divided by 400, or 55. Miss B completed the four minutes, and her pulse readings were 66, 57 and 53. She had a score of 68 (24,000 divided by 352).

Mr A was decidedly unfit: Miss B could be considered to be fairly fit, but needing to do better. Try the exercise yourself: if your score is 60 or less, you need to be much fitter. You can be described as only 'fair' if you score between 61 and 70, 'good' between 71 and 80, and 'very good' between 81 and 90. If you score 91 or more you are probably already an athlete in training.

Getting fitter

Now that you know how unfit you are, how do you start to be fitter? The principle is always to start slowly. If you have spent the last twenty or more years behind a desk, or the wheel of a car, or slumped in the armchair at home, your out-of-condition muscles will quickly complain at the change.

To start with, you don't need to jog or run, or to buy rowing machines or stationary cycles. Instead, make up your mind, in the first days, just to walk more. If you commute to work, walk to the station in the mornings and from the station at nights whenever the weather is reasonable. (Don't make up your mind to suffer in all weathers – you won't keep it up, and it may put you off the idea of walking.) If you normally take a bus or a tube train, get off a stop or two before your destination and walk the rest of the way.

Whenever you can, take the stairs, rather than the lift. Go by foot to any place within a mile of you, rather than take the car. Throw away the remote control on the television set, so that you have to get up to change the programme. Do, rather than watch, things in your spare time. Go swimming, or cycling, or walking, at weekends, rather than driving or staying at home. If you do stay at home, try gardening or fix those jobs around the house. Any activity is better than none.

Above all, do enough exercise to make yourself reasonably out of breath at least twice, and preferably three or four times, a week. If you think you will enjoy running, try it, but make sure that you have the right clothing and shoes, if you intend to run on pavements. Hard surfaces and the wrong shoes can badly jar ankle, knee and hip joints.

If you find that a particular exercise bores you, try something else. You are going to spend an appreciable time exercising in the future, and you will not keep it up if you don't really like it.

Don't take it too seriously, either. There are few people worse than an exercise bore, who is constantly talking about his times or speeds. In fact, don't buy a stop watch – competition and speeds are not part of the scene. The idea is to get away from stress, not to add to it. How long you spend on the exercise is probably more important than its severity. A 4 mile (6 km) walk will get your heart as fit as if you ran the same distance in half the time.

Exercise won't kill you. As long as you are sensible about starting, you don't need to consult your doctor before starting to get fit. There are even exercise routines for patients in heart failure, and they feel much the better for them!

Choose your exercise wisely. Don't opt for explosive exercises, such as weightlifting. The action of lifting weights or straining muscles while holding your breath is harmful, not beneficial. Doctors call this the 'Valsalva manoeuvre'. If you are not a trained weightlifter, it can cause a sudden drop in the amount of blood returning to the heart from the lower body. At best it will make you feel dizzy and faint, at worst you can quickly become unconscious. Explosive competitive sports like squash may also not be right for many people. Golf and tennis are more leisurely, and probably more acceptable.

If you are thinking of taking up a sport, then it is a good idea to have a few lessons from a professional first. It will not only give you an idea of how you will like it, but make it much easier for you to enjoy it. Few 'rabbits' survive for long in tennis or golf clubs unless they make very rapid progress in their skills.

Once you start your regular exercise, whatever it is, you are bound to have a few aches and pains as muscles are asked to do things that they have not done for years. As long as they disappear after resting, you can ignore them.

Don't overdo the exercise. If you start at a normal weight, and begin to lose a pound or two, then think again. You are either doing too much or not eating enough to replace the lost energy. It is no use replacing your heart attack risk with the problems of anorexia nervosa!

People can do too much, and become obsessed by exercise. James Fixx was probably one of these; he wrote that the best runners always look too thin. Being a beanpole has its disadvantages, and is not necessarily as good for you as being of normal weight. Of course, if you start by being overweight, losing the extra through exercise is a bonus, provided that you arrive at, and stay at, a normal weight for your height.

A point here: many people weigh themselves regularly. I don't recommend that, as it tends to focus on that one aspect, and can cause disappointment, if not despair, if the weight doesn't come off quickly. That is a mistake, because the exercise will alter your body shape, making you leaner and trimmer, without necessarily causing your weight to change much. The fat is replaced by more muscle tissue.

So instead of focusing on weight, follow your progress by looking in a long mirror. You will know from your shape and tone that you are improving, and that will boost your confidence rather than undermine it.

Daily exercise is all very well, but rest is important, too. The regular exerciser must have his rest periods, to let the muscles recover fully. So save one day a week for resting. Rest is important, too, at particular times of the day. Don't exercise until at least two hours after a main meal, or more than an hour after a small meal. Don't exercise after drinking alcohol.

If you are ill, don't try to keep up your exercise schedule, particularly if you have a virus infection such as influenza or a cold. As you begin to get better, however, start with a few easy exercises in the home – they will help your muscles to recover more quickly.

Never exercise until you are exhausted. Keep it moderate, so that you continue to enjoy it. Mixing your activities, too, will help you enjoy the new life more. Take your pick of golf, tennis, cycling, swimming, jogging, or simply walking the dog: do several of them, or even all of them, if you wish. The variety will give extra interest, and may widen horizons, too.

The benefits for your heart

Assuming that you do all this, what is in it for your heart? Regular exercise reduces the risk of, or postpones the onset of, a whole series of diseases, including arthritis, rheumatism, disc trouble, diabetes, high blood pressure, coronary disease, stroke and even depression and anxiety. If you are overweight it is the best way, eventually, to lose the flab.

People who exercise regularly are less likely to smoke and overeat, tend not to have high blood pressure, and have lower blood cholesterol levels. Their risk of a heart attack is much less than among those who take little exercise.

Exercising regularly also postpones the onset of old age, although it won't necessarily help you to live longer once you are old. It helps to 'compress' the final period of old age before death. You can tell an older person who has exercised throughout life by his or her straighter back, better neck movements, more mobile joints and more bulky musculature. Older people who are fitter feel less depressed and isolated from others.

This is particularly important for women. After the menopause, women's bones are particularly susceptible to osteoporosis, in which calcium, the mineral that provides strength to the bone structure, is lost gradually over the years; 12,000 women suffer broken hips every year in Britain alone because of their osteoporosis. Many of these fractures could have been avoided if only the women had taken regular exercise in the years leading up to the menopause.

Exercise strengthens bone by shunting calcium into it. Physically active women start their post-menopausal years with a much bigger 'bank' of calcium in their thigh and hip bones, so that any later loss of calcium will never be enough to cause the bones to weaken significantly.

It is never too late to start. From the early 1970s onwards, heart attack survivors have been encouraged to exercise as soon as they have recovered from the acute period. This has led to some astonishing success. One of the earliest proponents of exercise after heart attack was Dr Terence Kavanagh, who ran a Cardiac Rehabilitation Centre in Toronto.

He had encouraged his patients to start carefully, with a short walk, building slowly up to a slow jog for up to an hour at a time. Some of his patients suggested to him that they try a marathon. He was doubtful at first, but decided to encourage them. After careful training, all seven of his first group of patients finished the marathon without any ill-effects. According to James Fixx, they presented the good doctor with a trophy entitled 'Supercoach, the World's Sickest Track Club'!

No one suggests, of course, that every heart patient should be able to manage a marathon. In fact, the enthusiasm for marathons has died away since the early 1980s, rightly so, as it put too many untrained amateur would-be athletes at risk. Dr Kavanagh's club, however, shows that if people who have had heart attacks can do so well, exercise can offer so much more for all of us.

Once you start your new life of physical activity, how will you know if you are getting fitter? First, you will feel much fitter within yourself, physically, and you will be much more alert and happier, mentally. If you want to prove the benefit beyond doubt, however, try that Harvard Step Test again after one week of the new you! You will find your score going up dramatically: it will be easier to continue for the full four minutes, and your pulse rates will be much slower. Aim, eventually, for the mid-70 region, and keep yourself around there. You don't have to be an Olympic athelete to be fit and feel well.

6

Recognizing, and coping with, angina

Not so long ago people received the news of angina like a death sentence. It was accepted as the beginning of an inevitable progress towards a heart attack, and that, in turn, meant at best a life as an invalid, and at worst, sudden death.

If there is one message I would like to put across it is that these attitudes are outdated and should be forgotten. If you have angina you can take advice on self-management and medical treatment that will almost certainly allow you to live a normal, satisfying life. You may also need some form of operation to help your coronary circulation, but that is now so routine that it should raise no fears for anyone undergoing it.

Much of the fear can also be taken out of heart attacks. If you know a little about heart attacks, then you can help yourself through the worst period. You will understand why you are receiving the investigations and treatment, and will find it easier to follow your doctors' advice in the ensuing months and years. Remove the mystery, and you remove a lot of the fear.

Fear is a very destructive emotion, especially for the heart. It releases chemicals into the bloodstream that put up the blood pressure and cause the heart to race and demand more oxygen. It can stimulate the very event that you fear. Once you lose it, you will already have made the first step towards healing and full recovery.

This chapter concentrates on angina, what it is, how to recognize it, what to do about it yourself, and what your doctor is likely to do about it. Chapter 7 will do the same for heart attacks.

Angina – is it the heart, or something else?

Angina is simply the medical word for pain. Angina pectoris means pain in the chest, and the two words together have slipped into common usage as meaning heart pain.

Strictly that is not always the case. Many pains in the chest have no connection with the heart. Problems in the chest and upper back

63

that can produce pain include cramp or spasm in the chest wall muscles, or acid irritation flowing up from the stomach into the gullet. Often pain in the chest is no more than indigestion. Nerve irritations, as from shingles, or an inflamed lung surface, as in pleurisy, can also cause severe chest pain.

So, when you complain about chest pain, expect your doctor to ask searching questions about it: the answers you give will narrow down the possible causes. The first will be about the character of the pain: can you describe exactly what it feels like in simple terms?

The characteristics of heart pain are fairly clearly defined. If you describe it in one of the following ways, it will raise your doctor's suspicions:

tightness around my chest
a weight or pressure on my chest
constriction in my chest
an aching pain
a dull pain
a squeezing feeling
it's just sore
the chest is being crushed
there's a band round my chest
the tightness makes me breathless

If you describe the following your doctor will look for some other cause:

it's sharp
like a knife cutting me
it comes in stabs
it feels like a stitch
it's like needles in the skin
it shoots across my chest
it's worse if you press on it, or when I change position
I can walk around all day with it
it's there all day, even when I'm resting.

The next question is about where the pain is. The heart occupies a central-to-left position in the chest: heart pain, however, is not confined to the outline of the heart. It can spread up into the jaw, or down into an arm, into the back of the chest, or even into the upper stomach. It can feel as if it is vaguely in the centre of the chest, or towards the left side. However, it is rare for it to be entirely right-sided, without some part of it crossing the midline into the left.

An entirely right-sided pain is rarely cardiac in origin, unless you are one of a very rare breed, a 'mirror-image' twin. Some twins are born with all the main organs reversed in position, so that the heart tends more to the right, and the liver is on the left. When they develop angina it is on the right side.

The third question is when does the pain arise? Most angina starts with exercise. Physical effort brings it on, and resting relieves it. Your doctor will wish to know exactly how much exercise is needed to produce the pain, and how long it lasts when you rest.

Angina is graded according to how much exercise you can tolerate before the pain starts: from a few steps on the flat, through a brisk walk up a gentle slope, or climbing stairs, to running for a bus, digging, lifting weights, straining at the toilet, or making love. Don't hesitate to list *all* the times when you have noticed it: your doctor needs to know, and will not be embarrassed.

For a few people, angina comes on at rest or even wakes them out of sleep. *This is a serious sign, and needs urgent assessment in a specialist hospital department.* Prompt investigation in these cases can prevent an imminent heart attack.

The final question is – what do you do when the pain starts? Try to walk through it, or stop until it goes away? Whatever you have done in the past, the right course is to stop and rest. The pain is a sign that your heart needs more oxygen and must rest as much as it can to recover from its oxygen lack. So you must relax, preferably lie down, and wait for half an hour or so after the attack before moving again.

You may find that difficult to accept, especially if you are busy and want to get on with your work. If that is how you feel, then the next few paragraphs may convince you otherwise. They explain exactly what is going on in the heart during an angina attack, and why you must obey the advice.

The heart obeys a law as fundamental in biology as it is in the marketplace – supply and demand. The *supply*, in this case, is the supply of blood in the coronary arteries carrying oxygen and glucose to fuel the beating of the heart muscle. The *demand* comes from the need for the heart muscle to beat so that the heart can supply blood to all the other organs and tissues of the body. The more energy we expend, such as in physical exercise, or in digesting our food, or even in solving an intellectual problem, the more blood the heart needs to pump to the muscles, gut and brain, respectively.

Whenever the demand on the heart rises above the resting level, the coronary arteries must open up further and supply a better flow of blood to the myocardium. The heart beats faster, and more strongly, and needs to use up more oxygen and glucose to do so.

All this is very well catered for in the healthy heart, where the walls of the coronary arteries are smooth and elastic, and free of any obstruction. The problem starts when plaques of atheroma start to narrow and distort them. Such narrowed areas not only obstruct the free flow of blood, they are rigid, their elastic tissue being replaced by stiff, unyielding fibrous scars. They cannot open up to allow the extra blood through.

This means that the heart reaches a point at which the muscle beyond the narrowed segment of artery cannot get enough oxygen to fuel its contractions. This makes it impossible for the heart muscle to work efficiently, so that it becomes laden with acid residues of glucose. These chemical residues are the cause of the pain and other angina symptoms. When the heart muscle's demand for oxygen outstrips its supply by the coronary arteries, this is called medically *ischaemia*, a word that simply means a state of lack of blood. Coronary artery disease causing angina therefore has another name – 'ischaemic heart disease'.

Managing your own angina

Obviously there are two ways of reversing these effects. The first is to bring the work being done by the heart down to the resting level, so that the blood supply within the coronary arteries can again supply enough oxygen to the muscle. That means stopping all unnecessary activity, by resting.

The second is to try to improve the circulation in the coronary arteries, so that they will allow more blood flow through them.

There are three others, less immediately obvious options. You can make the blood that is flowing through the coronary arteries carry more oxygen. You can make the blood less viscous (less 'sticky'), so that it can flow more easily through the coronary system. And you can help to make the heart muscle itself contract more efficiently, so that it needs less oxygen to do the same amount of work.

We will take all these options one by one, showing how most people with angina can, by simple changes in their own behaviour, improve their symptoms.

The first step is to get into a routine with your angina. Whenever the pain starts, wherever you are, you must stop and rest completely, and remain at rest for 30 minutes. This gives your heart time to recover from that attack. Note the attack down, how severe it was, its relationship to exercise or exertion, how long it took to subside, and how soon you restarted your activities.

From then on your aim is to try, week by week, to improve your exercise tolerance. Do keep on exercising. Walking and swimming are good dynamic exercises that will improve the efficiency of the heart – but remember to stop as soon as you detect pain or discomfort.

The next step is to do all you can to keep your coronary arteries as wide open as possible. By now you will know that smoking narrows them, so you should stop all smoking – even one a day. Avoid other people's smoke, too. In a room full of smokers, you are unwillingly smoking one whole cigarette for every 20 smoked by the others. In today's social climate, you should not feel embarrassed to ask smokers nearby to stop or go elsewhere.

Next, embark on a long-term plan to reverse your atheroma, and therefore to reverse those narrowed sites in your coronary system – or at least prevent them from narrowing further still. It is never too late to start. The advice given on changing your eating habits to reduce your cholesterol levels applies just as much to you, if you already have angina, as to anyone else. The change in eating habits, by reducing your blood fat levels, will also appreciably reduce 'stickiness'.

Stopping smoking will also help the oxygen-carrying capacity of the red blood cells and the muscles of the heart itself; 15 per cent of the red cells of a 20-a-day cigarette smoker are clogged with carbon monoxide, and so cannot convey oxygen to the heart: stopping smoking gives the oxygen supply to the heart a welcome boost, *within a day of stopping*.

Washing out the carbon monoxide also improves the efficiency of the heart muscle cells by a similar extent, giving the supply–demand equation a double bonus. Remember that alcohol is a heart poison, except in very moderate doses, so always obey the rules mapped out in Chapter 4 on drinking.

Aspirin may also come in handy. There is good evidence, from trials of aspirin in doctors (22,000 in America and 5,000 in Britain) that aspirin every day may help to prevent angina and heart attacks in susceptible people. The doses used in the trials (one tablet every other day in the United States, and one every day in Britain) are small, but could well be even smaller. All that may be needed is half a tablet every day or on alternative days.

This small dose of aspirin helps to prevent the start of clotting in the bloodstream, and could help, like lowering cholesterol, to make the blood more fluid. At this dose, too, it is very unlikely to cause stomach upsets. If you have angina, you would be well advised to ask your doctor if you are suitable for this small dose aspirin treatment. Do not be tempted to increase the aspirin dose: this will not work, as at higher doses, the effect on clotting does not increase, but the side-effects will!

How your doctor will help

No matter how much you improve on your own, if you suspect you have angina, you *must* seek your doctor's help. Unfortunately, the severity of your symptoms does not correlate closely with the extent of the disease in your coronary arteries. Sometimes, the symptoms may be very minor, but there is extensive narrowing of all three main coronary arteries. This 'triple vessel disease' must be treated, often surgically, if a severe heart attack is to be averted.

There are even people who have symptomless 'silent' angina (except that they may feel vaguely unwell with exercise), and their condition is found by chance on a heart check-up. More complex still, many angina sufferers have 'silent' episodes of ischaemia, as well as their painful attacks, in which they should obey the same rules as for their known attacks. Obviously this can be difficult, as they have no warning that they should rest!

So, if you have pain or discomfort in the chest, at any time, you should seek medical advice. After ruling out other causes of the symptoms, and if there is even the remotest possibility that you have angina, you will be referred to your local hospital heart clinic for investigation.

Finding the causes of angina

The main aim of the clinic doctors will be to find the cause of the symptoms. Most of the time, in angina, this will be atheroma, affecting one or more of the three coronary arteries. However, there are a series of other causes, many of which are reversible, and all of which are treatable.

Prinzmetal angina. For example, a small group of angina sufferers have pain at rest, which disappears on exercise. This 'paradoxical' or 'Prinzmetal' angina (named after the doctor who first described it), is caused by the coronary arteries going into spasm, a form of cramp in the muscles within the coronary artery walls. As soon as Prinzmetal patients start to exercise, the coronary arteries relax, and the pain goes. This condition responds to 'calcium antagonist' drugs, that relieve spasm in these specific sites.

Aortic valve disease. Disease of the valve leading out of the left side of the heart, the 'aortic' valve, can also cause angina, in that the mechanism for 'sucking in' the blood to the coronary arteries, described in Chapter 2, is damaged. As the openings to the coronary arteries lie in the aorta, just above the valve, any distortion or disease of that valve can prevent free flow of blood into them. This form of angina is helped by replacing the diseased valve by a new one. Disease of the other valve in the left side of the heart, the mitral valve between the left atrium and the right ventricle, can also cause angina by putting too much strain on the heart. The answer here, too, is valve replacement surgery.

High blood pressure. High blood pressure may also cause angina, as the heart muscle thickens in response to the rising tension: the answer here is to lower the pressure by a combination of drugs and other lifestyle advice. (Readers who wish to know more might like to read my book *Living with High Blood Pressure*, also published by Sheldon Press.)

Anaemia. Anaemia is also a cause of angina; the blood contains too few red blood cells to carry enough oxygen to fulfil the heart's demands. Correcting the cause of the anaemia is the answer here.

Overactive thyroid. For many older women, angina can arise from an overactive thyroid gland. Too much of the thyroid gland's hormone, thyroxine, can make the heart beat too fast: correcting the tempo and slowing down metabolism provides the cure.

Abnormal rhythms. Finally, the angina may be caused by the heart going into an abnormal rhythm. In most people the heart beats at a steady rate, between 65 and 90 times a minute. In a few people the rate can become irregular, sometimes too fast, sometimes too slow. This can lead to difficulties for the heart muscle cells, in that they cannot recover sufficiently between beats before they get the signal to beat again. That can also affect the coronary flow of blood, so that the muscles lose their oxygen supply. The answer for such patients is to even out their pattern of heart beats; a whole series of new drugs has now been developed to do just this.

The heart unit – what to expect

You will have gathered from all this that the patient with angina needs extensive investigations to pinpoint the possible causes of his symptoms. The history and the examination will only take the doctors a short way along the road to the final diagnosis. If you have angina, you must expect to be asked to undergo exercise testing, special ECG tests and X-ray investigations, and perhaps coronary and heart catheter studies, in which the specialists can watch, directly, what is going on within your heart.

The exercise tests tell the specialist the level of exercise that your heart can stand before it begins to complain – in other words the severity of the angina. The ECG is a guide to which part of the heart is affected, and to what extent. The X-ray gives the dimensions of the heart, and shows how efficiently it is beating.

All this sounds frightening, but you should not let it worry you. In the modern heart units, everything is done to make sure that you are relaxed and unworried. The staff are very highly specialized, having concentrated on heart investigations for years, and knowing very well what entering a unit means for anyone.

I have visited many such units in Britain and Europe, all of them staffed by cheerful, kind and dedicated doctors and nurses who can make the most apprehensive patient feel happy and relaxed. The atmosphere is never one of 'doom and gloom' – it is much more of excitement and anticipation that their patients can be helped back to a normal life, with much to look forward to.

The first investigations are aimed at finding the underlying cause of the symptoms. The standard tests will rule out such problems as heart valve disease, high blood pressure, thyroid trouble and anaemia. They will be treated and, hopefully, this will cure the angina.

Most of the rest of the patients with anginal symptoms have atheroma. The next aim is to find out how serious it is, and the risk of a full-blown heart attack in the near future. That means trying to get as many details of how the heart is functioning at the time of an attack of angina.

The treadmill and Holter monitor

There are two main ways of doing this. First, you may be put on a 'treadmill'. This is a moving walkway, the speed and angle from the horizontal of which can be varied. The faster it moves and the steeper the incline, the more work it forces on the heart. While you use the treadmill, your heart is monitored by an ECG, which will show when the demand is beginning to outstrip the supply of oxygen – usually before you start to have pain. It will also show how much of the heart is affected, and which part of the heart. That helps to pinpoint which coronary artery or arteries are affected, and at which point of their distribution.

As a rough rule of thumb, if anginal pain, or ischaemic changes on the ECG, begins within two minutes of starting the standard treadmill exercise, then there is enough coronary disease for serious note to be taken. If you can go ten minutes or more without pain or silent episode, there is little to worry about.

Another approach, which can be used along with, or instead of, the treadmill, is to fit you up with a Holter monitor. This is a special portable, computerized, ECG machine, that you strap on to your chest for 24 or 48 hours. You then carry it on your person as you go about your normal life, waking and sleeping.

The Holter monitor records a continuous trace of your heart beats throughout that time, and can be programmed to 'pick up' all the episodes of ischaemia during that time, whether they caused pain or were symptomless. This gives a good idea of the burden of the angina, day and night.

Treadmill testing and Holter monitoring do detect those people at risk of a serious heart attack, so heart specialists now recommend that everyone with angina under the age of 65 years, regardless of the severity or mildness of the symptoms, should undergo them. For the over-65s, the decision to put them to such trouble depends on their general fitness and the severity of their symptoms.

Coronary angiography

If the treadmill and Holter tests show that you are having bouts of ischaemia, then the next step is coronary angiography. In this test, a small tube, or catheter, is fed from an artery in the leg or arm back up towards the heart. Dye is released into the openings of the coronary arteries, and the process watched under X-ray. This allows the cardiologist to examine the coronary branches, and therefore the circulation of the blood within the heart, in minute detail.

Coronary angiography pinpoints the sites of narrowing, where atheroma has reduced the flow of blood to the heart. This is vital information, because it directs the cardiologist to the next phase of your hospital visit – the decision on how to treat you.

Treating angina

Three choices are open for the angina victim. The first is non-surgical treatment, using drugs and advice on lifestyle. The second is bypass surgery, an operation in which the chest is opened and a vein is used to carry the much-needed blood around the narrowed areas of artery. The third is balloon angioplasty, a relatively new technique, in which the narrowed section of artery is 'blown up' by a small balloon around a very fine catheter. All three treatments will be explained here.

Medical treatments

Today, more and more angina sufferers are being offered one of the two surgical techniques; they are now highly successful in producing lasting relief from the symptoms. However, even patients who undergo bypass surgery or angioplasty may still have to take drugs, and all should obey the lifestyle rules outlined in Chapter 3.

There are three principal drugs for angina – the nitrates, betablockers and calcium antagonists. Nitrates act mainly by opening up the veins, all over the body, reducing the demand on the heart. They may also slightly open up the coronary arteries, improving the flow of blood through them.

Nitrates. The main advantage of nitrates is that, when placed under the tongue and allowed to dissolve, they work very quickly during an angina attack. If you are given them, your doctor will explain exactly how to use them. Under-the-tongue glyceryl trinitrate quickly puts the pain away: it then must be spat out, before other arteries, like those in the head, start to expand, too, causing a splitting headache!

Under-the-tongue nitrates can also be used to ward off an expected angina attack, as before climbing up a hill that you know can bring on pain.

Nitrates are also available in a spray which you place in your mouth, or in a patch, like a sticking plaster, which delivers the active ingredient through the skin. Many put the patch on their chests, but it would reach the heart just as quickly if placed anywhere on the torso. They seem to be useful in night pain or breathlessness, but not so effective against angina provoked by exercise or effort. Some nitrates, such as isosorbide dinitrate and mononitrates, are made up as tablets, to be swallowed. Side-effects of nitrates include headaches and flushing: if you can tolerate them for a few days, they usually disappear.

Betablockers. Betablocker tablets are the mainstay of most angina treatments. They reduce the demand on the heart, slowing the heart rate, lowering blood pressure and reducing the force of the heart beat. Each of these actions improves the balance between supply and demand.

The slowing of the heart beat on betablocker drugs can be dramatic: it may even drop down to around 45 or 50 per minute. This is nothing to worry about, as long as you feel well on the drug.

As with all active drugs, betablockers have side-effects. They include wheezing and heart failure in people whose hearts have already been damaged so patients are carefully selected before they are given them. Other, less serious, but sometimes annoying, side-effects, may include lethargy, bad dreams, a muzzy head, inability to concentrate. All betablockers produce cold feet, some to a lesser extent than others.

There are groups of betablockers with slightly different properties, so that if you find one does not suit you, you may be offered another. A list of their prescribed names include: acebutolol, atenolol, metoprolol, nadolol, oxprenolol, pindolol, propranolol, sotalol, and timolol. There are probably many more.

Calcium antagonists. Calcium antagonists, otherwise known as calcium entry blockers, are effective in both the 'Prinzmetal' angina due to spasm of the coronary arteries and in exertional angina. They work in several ways: they may lower the blood pressure by opening up the circulation in the legs and arms; they open the coronary arteries; and they improve the efficiency of the contraction of the heart muscle cells.

Calcium antagonists went through a bad time in the mid-1990s, because there was evidence that they might lead to sudden attacks of abnormal heart rhythm and to a higher risk of sudden death. That turned out to be linked to 'short-acting' calcium antagonists, the effects of which lasted only a few hours in each day, so that between times the control of the heart's beating mechanism was lost. All the newer preparations of calcium antagonists now exert their effects for 24 hours, and the problem has been solved. Current calcium antagonists include verapamil, amlodipine, felodipine, isradipine, lacidipine, lercanidipine, nicardipine, nifedipine and nisoldipine.

Side-effects of calcium antagonists include palpitations and flushing, but they are remarkably free from serious side-effects.

Surgical treatment

Angioplasty and bypass surgery have for the first time given doctors the opportunity to do something concrete about the supply, rather than the demand, side of the angina equation. The aim of both procedures is to increase the flow of blood to regions previously starved of oxygen because of narrowing of the coronary arteries.

If you are offered either of these treatments, you will first undergo a coronary angiograph, an X-ray which outlines the coronary arteries to determine exactly where the problem lies in the heart.

Angioplasty. Angioplasty is performed under sedation, but not under general anaesthesia, so carries less operative risk. It involves inserting a thin catheter (a flexible hollow tube) through an artery in the leg all the way back up the aorta into the affected coronary

74

artery, all the time under X-ray control. This is the easiest route for reaching the heart.

The tip of the catheter is passed through the narrowed segment of coronary artery. Just short of the tip the catheter forms a tiny balloon, which is inflated once it is exactly opposite the narrowed segment of artery. This compresses the area of atheroma, and widens the artery. After angioplasty, the flow of blood through that artery is usually multiplied many times over.

Doubts about angioplasty in the beginning have now been cast aside, as, after nearly 20 years of its general use, the success rates have been soaring. It has more than a 90 per cent success rate in coronary arteries, and many patients feel much better immediately after it has been done. Even angioplasty, however, has its problems: in about one case in 100, the catheter may block the vessel. This means that angioplasty must always be done in full operating theatre, so that an emergency coronary bypass operation can be done if necessary.

Bypass surgery. In bypass surgery a vein is taken from the leg or an artery from the inside of the chest wall, and inserted around the narrowed segment of coronary artery. The blood then flows through the new channel, rather than through the coronary artery, to the heart muscle beyond. The immediate result is much better flow of blood, and therefore glucose and oxygen, to the previously 'starved' area.

Bypass surgery is usually employed where there are multiple small blockages of one, two or three coronary arteries, and where the blockages are in vessels too small for angioplasty to be possible. Of course, it needs to be done under a general anaesthetic, and carries the risks, small as they now are, of any major operation.

More than two-thirds of bypass operations and angioplasties are still highly successful, with a wide open coronary circulation, six months later and beyond. The figures are improving all the time. Where they have been necessary, repeat angioplasties and surgery have been just as successful.

Many people have now enjoyed 20 years of very full active lives after their bypass operations and are coming up to their twentieth anniversary of their angioplasties. Their lives have been changed beyond their belief. The benefit cannot be put down entirely, however, to their surgery. The ones who really did best were those who were determined to change their lives.

They stopped smoking, controlled their drinking, changed their eating habits, exercised more, lost their excess weight, and adopted a wholly new style of life. Their hospital treatment offered them the chance to start life again – and they took it. This must be the lasting, definitive message for every angina patient.

Stents. Stents are tiny tubes, made up of a material that looks like a wire mesh. They can be placed in a narrowed segment of an artery using a catheter similar to the ones used for balloons. They are springy enough to keep open, and the open mesh system allows the new inside 'skin' of the artery to grow into it to make the smooth surface needed to keep the artery healthy. Many surgeons use stents instead of angioplasty or bypass in selected patients.

7

Heart attack!

Heart attacks, unlike angina, come out of the blue. They can as easily start in bed, or sitting watching television, as when playing squash, or losing your temper. They may strike when relaxing after a period of intense physical or mental stress. The attack that tragically ended the life of Jock Stein, the great Scotland soccer manager, happened just after his team scored the goal that put them into the Finals of the 1986 World Cup. His anxiety suddenly gone, he relaxed, and the heart attack started.

I can think of at least three heart attacks arising in similar circumstances:

- a 39-year-old professor who collapsed minutes after winning a gruelling game of league squash
- a 51-year-old doctor who died on the beach after rescuing a small child from drowning
- a 61-year-old businesswoman who had a heart attack half an hour after fighting off a would-be mugger in the street.

There may be a common link between them. In each case their blood pressures would have been very high in the period just before the attack, then dropped suddenly. This sudden change may have been just the stimulus needed to block off the flow of blood in one of the main coronary arteries. The heart rhythm may have been disturbed, and the chaotic beats that followed led to injury to the heart muscle.

In the case of two of the four – the football manager and the doctor, the damage was too great to survive. The professor and the businesswoman happily survived.

However, this is not the only pattern. People have fallen as if poleaxed while running for a bus, or suddenly pitched forward while reading, near bedtime. Heart attacks have taken people while asleep in bed or in an easy chair.

What does a full heart attack feel like? Survivors of the immediate attack describe the sensation very consistently. You feel a chest pain that is 'gripping' or 'like a vice' that goes on and on, unlike angina, even at rest. You may mistake it at first for indigestion, and try antacids and other 'stomach remedies' to clear it, unsuccessfully.

If you are already prone to angina attacks, you may delay asking for help in the belief that it is just another of the same. However, it is usually much more intense, and more persistent, and does not disappear with rest.

The centre of the pain is usually behind the breastbone, often higher, rather than lower, but it may spread from there to the jaw, neck, arms, back and into the upper abdomen, between the ribs. You become restless and anxious, and break out into drenching cold sweat. Onlookers see you as very pale and ill. You will know that this is something different from an angina attack. The moment that you realize this, ask for help.

If you are caring for a person who has suddenly entered this state, you must ring immediately for help. In most developed countries there are mobile coronary care services on an emergency telephone available to anyone. If you cannot immediately contact a doctor, then call that service. You will find that the response is fast and highly professional, with fully trained 'paramedic' ambulancemen and women who know how to deal with any heart problem.

In the unlikely event that neither doctor nor coronary ambulance is immediately available, then arrange to drive the patient to the nearest hospital with an emergency unit, avoiding all unnecessary noise, fuss or excitement.

The patient must be kept at rest all the time until he or she has professional help. In the meantime, the only medicine you should give is *one tablet of aspirin*: this will do no harm, and may just help by preventing further clotting in the coronary artery concerned.

If it is happening to you, try to remember that if you keep quietly at rest, and let everyone around you take all the strain, mental and physical, you have an excellent chance of survival. Don't try to organize yourself or to put last minute things in order – they can all wait until you come back, no matter how urgent they seem. Don't attempt to walk, or pack, or put on make-up or shave – just lie there and give your heart a chance to get into its resting state.

Absolutely, do not try to drive yourself! (That may seem unnecessary advice, but I would bet that every family doctor has witnessed the results of just such a decision by a very sick patient.) As for drugs, chew, then swallow one aspirin with a little water, but that is all. Have a list of any drugs you may be taking to show the ambulance or hospital staff.

Once you get into the hands of the ambulance men or emergency doctor, you will start to feel better, even before you are given anything more. Now is the time really to relax and lie back, because the risk to your life will rapidly diminish from now on, as the cardiac team take control.

Things will now begin to happen in quick succession. You will be linked up to machines to monitor your ECG and blood pressure. You will be given an injection to combat the pain and the anxiety. Blood tests will be taken to measure the extent of the heart muscle damage, if any; and you will be admitted to an intensive care ward, where every change in your condition will be monitored.

Visiting an intensive care ward when you are well can be frightening. Being a patient in one when you need the care is unbelievably reassuring and preferable to any other environment. So, if you are having a heart attack, don't hesitate to accept intensive care.

If, instead, you are caring for a heart attack victim at home, accept the advice that he or she should be admitted to intensive care. There is plenty of proof that the chance of survival is better, and that the quality of life after survival is now better after intensive care therapy.

What is it about intensive care that makes it so much better than home treatment? To understand the answer you must know what happens to the heart in an 'attack', and the complications that may follow. These complications must be reversed immediately – something that cannot be done at home.

Acute ischaemia, coronary thrombosis and myocardial infarction

Unfortunately, all branches of medicine are loaded with jargon. In the heart department, the 'buzz words' are 'acute ischaemic attack', 'coronary thrombosis' and 'myocardial infarction'.

In acute ischaemia, all the symptoms and signs of a full heart attack occur, but the incident stops just short of causing any real damage to the heart muscle. This is the mildest form of heart attack, and leaves you without any loss of heart tissue or scar.

An acute ischaemic attack may have been caused by a small thrombosis which blocked a coronary artery for a short time, but disappeared before there was time for it to cause heart muscle

79

(myocardial) damage. It may also have been caused by coronary artery spasm, although this is rarer. Either way, it causes the myocardium to go into a form of cramp. The treatment is to keep the patient at rest until the attack is past, usually within an hour or two, and then to start to find the underlying cause. That means following the same procedures as for angina, outlined in Chapter 6.

In coronary thrombosis, a branch of one coronary artery has become blocked, cutting off the blood supply to the heart muscle beyond the block. If it is not unblocked within a few hours, the affected muscle dies, and can no longer beat. The heart then loses that portion of its pumping action. The death of the muscle is referred to as myocardial infarction, often abbreviated to MI, the word infarction meaning destruction and degeneration.

The severity of the heart attack and the chance of a full recovery from the attack depends on the extent of the infarcted myocardium. In most people the area affected is relatively small, and there are few setbacks to a complete recovery. The infarcted (dead) heart muscle is cleared away by the body's natural healing processes, a scar forms, and the heart is usually well healed and functioning close to normal levels within less than six weeks.

The difficulties occur when the bulk of muscle deprived of its blood supply is larger. If a reliable blood supply is not restored within a few hours of the thrombosis, the death of such a large muscle mass leaves the heart in trouble. It may not be able to pump efficiently, and there may also be extensive damage to the network of electrical fibres that coordinate the pumping action of the heart (see Chapter 2). What remains is a pump that is only partially efficient even at the best of times, and that is prone to abnormal rhythms because of its electrical pathway disturbances.

It is precisely this sort of complication that intensive care units (ICUs) have been designed to avoid, if possible. If patients can reach their local ICU within the first hour or so of their attack, they now have a reasonable chance of survival with the minimum of permanent heart damage. The whole purpose of ICUs is to stop any further damage to the heart and, if possible, to reverse the damage that has already occurred.

Heart tests

The potential extent of the heart damage can be predicted, soon after entering the unit, from two tests.

Electrocardiogram

The electrocardiogram shows very specific changes which not only help to assess the amount of muscle damage, but its site. It can determine whether the infarct affects the left or right chambers, or the upper or lower surfaces of the heart.

Testing for enzyme levels

The second test involves a simple blood test for enzyme levels. These enzymes are released from dying muscle cells into the blood stream: the levels reached directly reflect the amount of heart muscle damage by the infarction. High enzyme levels and big ECG changes suggest a difficult recovery period; small changes in both suggests guarded optimism about the outcome.

Assessment of the ECG findings together with the enzyme test results, therefore, gives the doctors a good guide to the extent of the heart muscle loss, which sector of the heart is affected, and the prospects for recovery to good health.

For most MI patients, these tests are all that are needed to make the diagnosis and to form the basis for treatment. A small minority, however, need more tests. Some of them may be more seriously ill than the ECG or enzymes suggest, others may be sliding into 'heart failure', a condition in which the heart beat is not strong enough or efficient enough to maintain the circulation.

Ventriculography

These patients may need a technique called ventriculography to determine exactly where the fault lies. This involves a special X-ray (a *contrast ventriculogram*) or radioisotope system (a *scintigram*) under either of which the radiologist can watch the movement of the heart with each beat, and examine damaged areas in detail. That allows any possible surgery to be planned very meticulously in advance.

In some severe cases, the heart wall can be so damaged that it thins out to form a balloon-like weak spot. Nowadays this 'aneurysm' can be removed: the remaining heart muscle can then become an efficient pump again, and add years of valuable and worthwhile life to a person who would otherwise have died. Ventriculography is used to identify this type of damage.

Ventriculography involves either swallowing a tasteless liquid or receiving a small injection; the only other demand on the patient is that he or she lies still while the cardiac team watch the X-ray or television screens.

Treating a heart attack – the first few hours

Of course, in the first few hours after a heart attack, the intensive care team is not just waiting around for the test results: your treatment starts from the moment you enter the unit. It has two immediate aims – to remove any pain and shock, and to minimize the amount of heart muscle damage.

The first is achieved by giving pain relief and sedation. For most people that means injections of morphine or some similar narcotic drug. That has the double advantage of easing anxieties and calming the heart and circulation.

The second aim is achieved by doing everything possible to get rid of any clot that may be blocking a coronary artery. This was, of course, the purpose of the aspirin tablet given before the admission to hospital. It will be followed, either in the emergency ambulance or as soon as you enter the unit, by injections of 'thrombolytic' (clot-dissolving) agents. Heparin or warfarin, 'anticoagulant' drugs that prevent further clots from forming, will probably be added.

If this combination of treatments is given to full heart attack victims in the first six hours of their attack, they have a much better chance of survival than if their admission to hospital is delayed, or if they are kept at home.

For most MI victims, this acute period is the vital one. Once they have survived the first day, the road to full recovery is steady and uneventful. They are asked to get out of bed within a few days, and the vast majority go home within seven to ten days. Many need no further drug treatment, except, perhaps, the betablockers, calcium antagonists or nitrates described in Chapter 6 (pages 63–76).

Arrhythmias

For a small number of MI patients, however, the ICU is a real life-saver. For them, the heart attack may have damaged not only the heart muscle, but the complex network of nerve cells that coordinate the heart beat. This can lead to *arrhythmias*, in which the heart can suddenly lose its regular, steady rhythm, and burst into runs of beats that are slower, faster, or much more irregular than normal.

This abnormal form of heart beat may simply be an inconvenience – the palpitations felt by some people after drinking too much coffee is an example. After an MI, however, it can be life-threatening. This is why every patient admitted because of a heart attack spends the first few days 'wired up' to an ECG monitor, which will sound an alarm at the first evidence of an arrhythmia.

The peak time for such arrhythmias is the first 48 hours after the attack. Sometimes it is the recovery of the heart muscle, when the blood supply starts to return to it after an artery is unblocked, that stimulates the arrhythmia. The ICU staff are very well aware of this danger period of 'reperfusion'. They are prepared for it with an armoury of 'antiarrhythmic' drugs.

They are also trained to use the *defibrillator*, an electrical machine used to stimulate the 'fibrillating', or shivering heart back into a normal rhythm. This shivering rhythm is the most dangerous of all the arrhythmias, in that, untreated, it *always* leads to death.

Arrhythmias have to be reversed within minutes, and sometimes within seconds, if lives are to be saved. For this reason alone, if I were to have a coronary, I would opt for ICU admission, at least for the first week.

Home is only comfortable and reassuring if you don't need professional help immediately to hand. It is impossible to predict, from the severity of the initial attack, who will develop an arrhythmia. It can be stimulated by even the most minor MI, so that there is really no case for keeping anyone with a proven heart attack at home.

Heart failure and heart block

Other complications of a heart attack are heart failure and heart block. In heart failure, the heart beat cannot generate enough power to maintain adequate blood flow to all the regions of the body. Fluid builds up in the tissues and the lungs, and the patient becomes weak, breathless and swollen.

Heart failure is usually a sign of relatively severe myocardial damage. If it occurs in the first few days, the action of the heart can be helped by extra pumps attached to the circulation, programmed to beat in coordination with the heart beat. This can only be a temporary measure, until the heart recovers as fully as possible from the damage. Drugs to improve the heart beat and to remove the strain from the heart will help to some extent in the initial period.

Many patients do recover from this form of heart failure, and go on to leave hospital and enjoy good health. For a minority, however, the cause of the failure is the extent of the damage to the heart – and this is too great to allow recovery. For these people, heart transplant is the only option. It is not an easy option: transplant waiting lists are long, and priority must be given to the young. Life after transplant is much preferable to the alternative, but it also has its problems.

Waiting for a transplant involves much personal care from doctors, nurses, physiotherapists, and above all, family. It means the need for support for the failing heart using drugs. The patient needs a balanced personality, a full understanding of what lies ahead, and acceptance that it will not be easy.

A successful transplant is like being reborn. Many patients are able to do things they have not done for years: they enjoy life to the full. However, the price to be paid is a lifetime of watching for infection and rejection. As treatments of both these complications improve, more and more heart transplant patients are living long, successful and fulfilling lives.

Heart block may be another complication of heart attack, although it can arise out of the blue in an otherwise normal heart. In heart block, the electrical message to the heart muscle to contract does not pass as it should from the upper chambers, the atria, to the lower chambers, the ventricles. The ventricles therefore decide to beat at their own rate, which is usually too slow for comfort or for the needs of the circulation.

The answer to heart block is usually a *pacemaker*, which stimulates the ventricles to contract at the desired rate. Pacemakers are inserted under the skin of the chest, in a minor operation; leads from the battery stimulate the heart to beat at the rate set in the pacemaker.

Most MI patients who need pacemakers only do so for the first week or so. The heart usually slips back into a normal rhythm itself, and the pacemaker can be removed. For the small minority who need more permanent pacemakers, they are now so small and so convenient that their wearers can virtually forget them until their annual consultant appointment. Today's pacemakers are even programmed to increase and decrease their rates of 'firing' to cope with their wearer's needs.

From this description of the modern management of heart attacks, it is reasonable to be optimistic about the future of anyone who reaches the relative security of an intensive care unit. Most patients who reach it alive come out of it alive and looking forward to a worthwhile quality of life.

It must still be stressed, however, that around one-third of all heart attack victims die in the first few hours of their first attack – before they reach the emergency ambulance or hospital. Of those that reach hospital six hours or more after the onset of their attack, around one in five will die some time in the next year from a further attack or from heart failure. This figure improves to one in six if the hospital treatment starts within six hours, and to one in eight if it begins within one hour.

These figures, from a study of 11,712 Italian heart attack patients, reported in 1987, suggest that there are two lessons to be learned. The first is that time must never be lost in moving people with suspected heart attacks into hospital – the sooner thrombolytic (clot-dissolving) treatment is started the more chance there is of long-term survival.

The second is that leaving hospital well after your heart attack is only the first step towards a new life. Your prime aim should then be to ensure that you do not have another attack, and that you can look forward to a long and happy life ahead. How to try to achieve this is the subject of Chapter 9.

8

Women and heart disease

Coronary artery disease is now the commonest cause of death in women in many countries, including Britain and the United States. In the United States, it kills proportionately more women than men. This is mainly because in women the risk of heart attacks rises steeply after the menopause. Before the age of 65 heart attacks are twice as common in men as in women: by 65 the sexes have an equal risk. In the over-80s and beyond, heart attacks are much more common in women.

However, heart attacks do occur in much younger women: a quarter of the deaths from myocardial infarction in women under 65 happen to women under 45. So women of all ages should be aware of their risks, and how to lower them. Their doctors also need to be more aware of them. For there is good evidence that many heart problems in women of all ages are going undiagnosed, and that women are suffering unnecessarily because of it. Three papers published in the *British Medical Journal* (3 September 1994) make that clear.

Dr Karen Clarke and her colleagues of Nottingham University studied the cases of men and women admitted to their hospital with suspected heart attacks (myocardial infarctions) in 1989 and 1990. The differences between the sexes were remarkable: of those who actually had infarctions, the women took longer to arrive in hospital, were less likely to be admitted to the coronary care unit, and less likely to receive anti-thrombotic treatment such as aspirin and streptokinase. They had more severe infarcts, were more ill, and were slightly more likely to die during their hospital stay than the men. They were less likely to be given aspirin and betablockers as preventive medicine after they went home.

Dr Clarke concluded that 'overall, women with ischaemic heart disease seem to be receiving a less than fair deal'. Her feelings were confirmed by Dr Paul Wilkinson of the London School of Hygiene and Tropical Medicine, and his team. They followed women and men admitted to a coronary care unit in London from 1988 to 1992. In the six months after admission to hospital 63 per cent of the women and 76 per cent of the men survived with no further cardiac events. The overall survival rates were 70 per cent for the women and 84 per cent for the men. Although the women were on average older than the men – as they were in Dr Clarke's patients – the difference in survival was not due to the difference in age. When women and men of the same age were compared, the women were more likely to succumb from their infarction.

In the past, the blame for the relatively high number of women dying of heart attacks has been placed on the fact that they are more likely to have high blood pressure and diabetes. But even when Dr Wilkinson's team removed these illnesses from their analysis, proportionately more women died from their attacks than did the men.

The major loss of life among the women occurred in the first 30 days. This was attributed to the fact that they had had less vigorous treatment for their heart attacks than their male counterparts. Dr Wilkinson thus concluded 'effective strategies must be developed to protect women during this early period'.

Research by Philip Hannaford, Clifford Kay and Susan Ferry of the Manchester Research Unit of the Royal College of General Practitioners showed that many of the consultants operated a policy of not giving older patients thrombolytic treatment (anticlotting therapy such as streptokinase) – and women tended to fall into the older category.

The differences between the sexes do not end at the provision of acute treatment. In an American study headed by Dr M. A. Pfeffer, although angina was the same in both sexes, twice as many men as women were given angiography and coronary artery bypass grafts. In yet another study, by J. N. Tobin and colleagues, men with abnormal heart movement scans were ten times more likely to have angiography, and for a given coronary abnormality were four times more likely to have coronary bypass surgery than women with the same degree of disease.

So not only are women losing out on initial care of their heart attacks, they may also be faring worse than men in later corrective treatment of their coronary arteries.

What can women do about this? It is true that women who develop heart attacks tend to be older, and that they are more at risk from heart attacks if they have high blood pressure, diabetes and heart failure. These risks must be controlled. If you are female and have high blood pressure or diabetes (or both – they often go together), you should do all you can to make sure that they are kept under strict control.

For high blood pressure that means taking the correct anti-high blood pressure treatment and having regular (i.e. monthly) blood pressure checks. For diabetes that means strict control of weight (avoiding excess poundage like the plague) and of blood glucose levels and insulin dosage. High-fibre diet, multiple daily doses of insulin, a daily diary card of blood glucose measurements and monthly attendance at your general practitioner diabetes clinic are essentials.

Heart attacks are less common in premenopausal women than in men of the same age group because they are partially protected against heart attacks by their female sex hormones – particularly by oestrogen. When oestrogen is lost after the menopause their heart attack rates shoot up.

So why not give oestrogens after the menopause, as hormone replacement therapy (HRT), to keep the heart attack rates low? In May 2002, the British Heart Foundation (BHF) reviewed in its Factfile for UK general practitioners its thoughts on HRT and heart disease. It seems the jury is still out on whether HRT helps reduce heart problems for older women. The BHF admits that heart disease is reduced up to 40 per cent in women using HRT. However, they are generally healthier in the first place than women not on HRT, so that their better health in the long run may simply be due to bias in their selection.

We are still waiting for the results of two long studies (one American and one international) in normally healthy women, some using HRT and some not. Both aim to see if using HRT prevents heart attacks. Two American trials in women who started on HRT after they were known to have heart disease have not shown that HRT has improved their disease. Named the Heart and Estrogen/progestin Replacement Study (HERS) and the Estrogen Replacement and Atherosclerosis (ERA) trial, these two trials are continuing.

My own feeling is that women should take HRT if they feel better on it, and not to start it as a way of avoiding heart attacks.

Worries that HRT may increase the risk of breast cancer have now been addressed by figures from a host of studies. In women using it for long periods, it seems that their risk of breast cancer rises by 2.3 per cent per year. This is just the same as if they were delaying the onset of the menopause (there is a higher risk of breast cancer in women whose periods stop at later ages than the average). The risk falls again on stopping HRT. This should not stop women taking

HRT unless they have had close relatives with the disease, but they should have regular breast examinations when on HRT.

HRT is not all bad news. It does have advantages. A review of 29 studies of HRT, quoted by the same BHF Factfile, reported that HRT in women taking it for menopausal symptoms (such as flushes, depression, difficulties with intercourse, and osteoporosis) improved their verbal memory, reasoning and the speed with which their muscles worked. There is preliminary evidence that it might stave off dementia, but the proof of that awaits the results of yet more trials.

One risk in men – very high blood fat (cholesterol) levels – may not apply in the same way to women. Younger women naturally have higher blood cholesterol levels than men of the same age, but most of the cholesterol is in the form of the 'good' HDL type. So no woman should rely on a total blood cholesterol count to assess her heart attack risk. The cholesterol *must* be divided into the different cholesterol fractions, such as LDL and VLDL, the 'bad' types, and their proportion to HDL should be studied. Only if there is something seriously amiss should cholesterol-lowering drugs or diets be undertaken, and only then under specialist supervision.

Of course, the other major risk for heart attacks is smoking. Younger women are apparently turning more to cigarettes than did previous generations. The increasing habit may reflect stresses socially or at work, but the cigarette companies are certainly targeting young women with their advertising. Women also use cigarettes to keep fashionably slim – as they destroy their appetite. The fact that smoking also destroys their complexion, their looks, their lungs, and eventually their hearts, does not seem to matter so much.

For women who smoke, the facts are simple. Dr Graham Jackson, consultant cardiologist at Guy's Hospital, London, puts them starkly:

- premenopausal smokers have three times the rate of infarction of non-smokers;
- women smoking more than 40 cigarettes a day increase their risk 20-fold;
- the combination of smoking with diabetes is particularly hazardous, adding steeply even to these risks;
- smoking and the newer contraceptive pills do not apparently increase the severity of coronary heart disease, but oral contraceptive users should not smoke (as it does increase the risk of thrombosis in other sites, such as the pelvis, legs and brain).

Women who undergo coronary artery bypass surgery have a slightly higher risk of complications afterwards than men, but this is probably because by the time they reach the surgeon's table their coronary disease is more advanced than that of the men. They also have naturally narrower coronary arteries. However, the results of today's coronary artery grafts are now just as good for women as for men, and the risk is small. For women with angina, who have not had an actual infarct, the long-term outlook is better than for men.

Dr Jackson also comments that once diagnosed as having coronary artery disease, women are less likely to be referred to, or take up the offer of, rehabilitation classes. They tend to be more depressed, anxious, and even to feel more guilt about their illness, than men. He asks for rehabilitation courses to be tailored specially for women and their different needs.

'Women', said Dr Jackson, writing for doctors in the *British Medical Journal*, 'are different – but not that different. Although women with coronary artery disease may be more difficult to diagnose and manage than men, it is a challenge that we (doctors) and they must rise to.'

'An equal opportunity killer needs equal opportunity management.' I wholeheartedly agree. Doctors have been alerted by the series of *British Medical Journal* articles to the need to treat women with heart disease more vigorously. It is now time that you, women yourselves, recognized more fully that you are at risk. Do not ignore that pain in the chest. Do not smoke – at all. Do have regular health checks, and, if you have high blood pressure or diabetes, *do* take care to control it properly. Do try to keep to a normal weight – not overweight, but not too thin. Most models in women's magazines are far too thin. Some look anorexic, and that too causes heart disease. Be just about the right weight for your height, and you won't go far wrong.

9

After the attack

If there has been one theme that has taxed the medical imagination over the last quarter of the twentieth century, it has been how best to help people who have just recovered from a heart attack. Subjects have ranged from drugs to prevent a second attack, to diets and exercises to reduce blood fat levels, and ways to lower the other risk factors such as smoking and drinking.

General practitioners like myself, while appreciating the fact that such research is vital – and appreciating the hard work put into it – should be forgiven if they feel, sometimes, that the everyday worries of the patients are being overlooked in all this science.

So, before going into the details of the best ways to keep alive for the longest time after a heart attack, I feel this is a good place to review just how most recovered heart attack victims feel about themselves.

How are you feeling?

If you have just had a heart attack, you are probably physically unfit, partly because you took little exercise before your attack, and partly because your recent enforced rest has weakened your muscles further.

You will probably be depressed. This is understandable, as your life has been threatened, and you worry about your next attack. You probably have noticed an occasional 'missed beat', or a minor left-sided chest pain, and they have frightened you. You may have found that you are having angina at an exercise level well below that before the attack, or that you get easily breathless on relatively slight exertion.

Then, with this in the background, you find that you cannot face the return to work that is looming ahead. This is just as true for the sedentary office employee as for those doing heavy manual labour. Most jobs need physical fitness, and to be physically fit, you need an underlying mental attitude combining self-confidence with tranquillity about the future and lack of fear. Lying awake at nights, and sitting around the house all day, three or four weeks after a major heart attack, do not promote this desirable mental state!

The fact is that many patients feel forgotten in the weeks after they leave hospital. No matter how well-meaning their family doctors and nursing care, it is bound to be much less intensive than the hospital environment. The constant hospital round of doctors, nurses, physiotherapists, the visits to X-ray, and the company of other patients give little time for introspection.

At home it is introspection time all day – and much of the night! You may have a daily visit for a while from the district nurse and a twice weekly doctor's visit. With luck you may even be seen by a physiotherapist. Sadly, the arrangements for follow-up at home vary from place to place, and are rarely ideal. It is easy to become despondent.

In fact, most men and women recovering from a heart attack are much healthier than they think they are. They naturally tend to look on the black side, when they could be much more active, physically and mentally. Most people recover from their myocardial infarction to a good performance level, measured by treadmill and bicycle tests; it is their mental attitude that tends to hold them back. Half of those not back at work six months after the attack are suffering from cardiac neurosis (excessive anxiety about their heart), rather than physical disability.

Rehabilitation

The key to bringing 'heart' patients back to normal life, therefore, is rehabilitation, both physical and mental. The process should start in hospital, where you are encouraged to be mobile as early after the attack as possible, and to be optimistic about your future physical abilities. Video sessions showing how former patients have recovered, and visits from former patients, are extras that many hospitals are now providing.

Within three to four weeks of your attack, or five or six weeks after bypass surgery or angioplasty, you will be introduced to a scheme of gradually increasing exercise, planned for you by your physiotherapist and doctors. The amount you will be asked to do is based on your performance on a careful treadmill or bicycle test, monitored by ECG to assess the extent of any residual heart problem.

If this test finds that your angina is worsening, or that there is a tendency to arrhythmia or heart failure, then you will be sent back for further treatment to your hospital physician. If not, you can start on the exercise programme.

The aim of the exertion is to speed up your heart rate to 85 per cent of your 'predicted maximum'. For most people this turns out at around 195 minus your age, so that if you are 50 years old you would expect to exercise enough to raise your pulse to 145 beats per minute. This is not because you should not go further, but because there is no need to; you will achieve as much benefit by keeping under the limit as by going all out.

The kind of exercise matters. It should emphasize movement, rather than power. Coronary rehabilitation groups in Britain, most of which are based in hospital physiotherapy departments, usually employ circuit training. This mixes stationary cycling with stepping up and down, jogging on a mini-trampoline, and a series of arm and leg exercises using light dumbbells.

This variety is important, not only because it helps avoid boredom, but because it spreads the exertion across a range of muscle groups, 'limbering up' the whole body for eventual return to work and other activities. Cycling and jogging are popular with some groups, but they all feel that a warm-up with easy callisthenics and a 'warm-down' with a game – preferably non-competitive – leads to enthusiasm for a return visit. The whole session lasts for between 20 and 30 minutes.

You should attend training sessions like these three or four times a week: twice a week is the minimum. At this rate, your fitness will improve very quickly; trying to do more will be of no extra benefit and carries risks of muscle injuries or, if your heart is not quite back to normal, of inducing arrthythmias.

Each person attending one of these cardiac rehabilitation groups has different needs and abilities. The rule is to start off with very light exercise, and build up over succeeding sessions, increasing the exercise load according to the heart rate from the previous session. Partners such as spouses should be encouraged to attend and join in; this gives them an idea of how much exercise can be done, and may stop well-meaning but overprotective care at home.

For the first three weeks or so, all the exercise sessions must be supervised by a professional. From then on, you will be encouraged to do home exercises as well, on the same pattern, and keeping your pulse rate to that 85 per cent of maximum. The 'circuit' can include jogging on the spot, stepping up and down two steps and swinging 3 kg dumbbells. It should then extend to outdoor walks, of, say, one to two miles ($1\frac{1}{2}$ to 3 km), which can be further extended to a jog in two or three more weeks.

The length of most hospital-organized rehabilitation varies from around six to twelve weeks, depending on the resources available and the numbers of patients. It takes about this time to sort out the different needs of those with little or no heart damage from those with need for more care. It also gets the patients used to regular exercising, and to get into the frame of mind that exercise like this is for ever, and not just to get over that particular attack.

Rehabilitation works on several levels. It brings people back to fitness as quickly and pleasantly as possible. It gives them confidence that they can return to a full life – often in a fitter state than they were before their attack. The exercise itself, combined with the new-found confidence, helps to dispel the depression and anxiety that naturally comes with the realization that you have had a heart attack. The new attitudes to life are a bonus, as are the new friends you meet in the group.

The friends are a help in another way. They, like you, will be trying to give up all the bad habits that led to their heart attack. They will be trying to lose weight, to give up smoking, to change their eating habits in the right direction – often all at once. Tension, anxiety and depression all have to be faced, openly. It is much easier to do all this along with others in the same boat than to try to go it alone.

Cardiac self-help groups often carry on meeting long after the hospital has had to wish them goodbye. They become 'self-help clubs' in which they share in their exercise, recreation and friendship. They can be a powerful source of support in times of need.

Many general hospitals provide coronary rehabilitation programmes for their heart attack patients. Dr H. J. N. Bethell, a general practitioner from Hampshire, England, described the one set up by his local hospital, in a *British Medical Journal* article in 1988 (297, 120). He calculated then that it trained about 100 patients back to health a year, at a cost of £53 per rehabilitated patient. This is less than the cost of half a day in hospital.

These economics must surely be worth it. No hospital should be without a rehabilitation programme: if yours has none, perhaps a little pressure on the authorities by the patients and their relatives may help to change their point of view!

Back to normal

What about returning to normal activities? Questions that are bound to arise are:

● *When will I be my normal self again?*

Most people should be fit to return to a normal, active life in under four weeks from leaving hospital. If you aim for that, and for a return to work in, say, three months, you will be surprised how good you feel about your new approach to life. Many patients have looked back on their heart attacks, finally, not as a terrible event in their lives, but as an opportunity to take stock, and to change for the better. This attitude cannot be bettered.

● *What are my chances of another attack?*

Much of that depends on you, and whether you take heed of the main risk factors of smoking, high cholesterol levels and high blood pressure. Stop smoking, eat correctly, exercise according to your rehabilitation programme and, if you have high blood pressure, follow your doctor's advice on treatment for that. Do all these things, and your chance of a second attack recedes into the distance.

● *Can I start gardening?*

Gardening is an excellent form of exercise. Provided you take it gradually, and keep within your fitness level, few gardening tasks will be beyond you. Unless you are extremely fit, and have been given the all-clear from your consultant, digging in heavy soil is out. The same goes for lifting and pushing a heavy wheelbarrow, or shovelling deep snow. In six years in one general practice there were three sudden deaths in men who had had previous heart attacks. Two were found stretched over their wheelbarrows, and one beside his garden path newly cleared of snow.

• *Will I ever drive again?*

It is very rare for people to have to stop driving, unless they have regular angina attacks. Most heart attack survivors return to driving within three months.

• *What about sexual intercourse?*

Lovemaking is not only good exercise, it would be cruel and even counterproductive to forbid sex, with all the extra anxieties and stresses that it would produce. Nevertheless, it is best to take it relatively easy for the first few weeks after leaving hospital.

Drugs and oily fish!

If you are recovering from a heart attack, you will also have heard, if not from your doctors, from other patients who have travelled the same road, about the various ways in which your risk of future infarctions can be lowered still further.

Betablockers

The first to be publicized was the use of betablocker drugs. As explained in Chapter 6, betablockers reduce the heart rate and the force of the beat, reducing the demand for oxygen. Trials first in Norway, then in other parts of Europe and North America, showed that if heart attack survivors took a small betablocker dose every day, routinely, there was less long-term risk of early death from another heart attack.

This led, for a while, to their routine prescription to virtually all patients recovering from heart attacks. Those who had asthma, heart failure, or who found the side-effects of the drug too much, did without. Until recently, most doctors gave betablocker agents to heart attack survivors unless there was a good reason not to do so. Many still give them, and on the evidence it is with good reason.

Aspirin

The second series of major trials to show that a drug would reduce the risk of death after a heart attack involved aspirin (see also page 80). Aspirin was tested because it prevents the formation of clots in small arteries. Several of the trials involved a combination of aspirin with another drug, dipyridamole, which also lowers the chance of

96

bloot clotting. Aspirin, with or without dipyridamole, did lower the death rate after heart attacks.

The news of the aspirin results led to its almost universal adoption for the long-term prevention of heart attacks, especially in patients who had already had one attack. At half a tablet a day, now the recommended dose for its anticlotting activity, it is very cheap and almost free of side-effects, two considerable advantages over betablockers.

Some doctors have switched from betablockers to aspirin; others have decided, on the 'belt and braces' principle, to prescribe both. The combination should do no harm, although there is no proof that the extra treatment will give extra benefit. Should you worry if you are not given a prescription for either? On balance I would say yes, if only because the evidence that they prevent second and further attacks is now so good. Aspirin, in the current low dose of 75 mg a day, is probably a reasonable self-help medicine.

The oily fish diet

In the latter half of 1989, the cardiac news was all about oily fish. In 1983, the British Medical Research Council (MRC) set up a study to find out if men who had had heart attacks could reduce their risk of death or a second attack by changing their diet.

Three diets were chosen:

- a reduced fat intake, increasing the ratio of polyunsaturated to saturated fat.
- an increase in oily fish consumption such as mackerel, herrings, kippers, trout, salmon, sardines and pilchards.
- an increase in cereal fibre, such as wholemeal bread, and bran.

More than 2,000 men under 70 recovering from heart attacks were allocated to advice on one, two, or all three diets or to no advice at all, making eight groups. They were then followed for five years, the researchers doing their best to confirm at intervals that they were sticking to the advice given.

Interestingly the men found it easier to cooperate with the 'oily-fish' and the 'increased fibre' advice than with the change in food fats.

The report of the trial, published in the *Lancet* in 1989 (Burr, M. L. et al., 298, 920), was astonishing. Within two years of their heart attacks, the half of the men given the oily fish advice had many fewer deaths (94) than the half who did not (130). When all the calculations were made, the oily fish appeared to have reduced the numbers of deaths by as much as 29 per cent. Increasing cereal fibre did not confer benefit, and the advice on fats was not taken, so that its effect could not be measured.

These results have caused a considerable stir among the columns of the *Lancet*. The trial and its results have been criticized, and speculations on how oily fish could have been so beneficial have been rife. There has been considerable argument about the possible connections between the oily fish diet and the lack of heart attacks in fishing communities such as the Japanese and the Greenland Inuit (Eskimo).

It is too early to be sure whether this reduction in deaths was a real effect, or was a quirk of that particular trial. However, survivors of heart attacks will do themselves no harm if they try the fish diet themselves. All it needs, apparently, is for them to eat a helping of oily fish three times a week in place of their usual meals.

What all this boils down to is that survivors of heart attacks can do much to help themselves to an active, satisfying life. The cornerstones of that life are exercise, sensible eating, perhaps a betablocker and/or an aspirin a day, and possibly an oily fish meal three times a week. Most of all, however, it needs belief in themselves, so that they feel whole again, and not some sort of cripple, waiting for the next catastrophe. Spouses can help greatly by encouraging them with kindness to comply with their doctors' advice – without appearing to nag. If that is the main message coming out of this book, then it has achieved its aim.

10
Managing heart disease – an update

Many of the trials of new treatments of heart disease that were started in the 1980s and continued into the first half of the 1990s have been completed, published and reviewed by panels of experts. These reviews have been the basis of guidelines for doctors to use in people at risk of, or in the process of having, a heart attack.

A 'buzz' phrase in medical treatment is 'evidence-based medicine'. There are several reasons for this. Treatment costs are rising steeply, and doctors must be able to justify treatments by comparing the costs of prescribing them with the benefits to be gained from them. We suspect, too, that the perceived benefits from many traditional treatments have no real basis in fact. So all current treatments, new and old, are now subject to detailed analysis, and to randomized controlled clinical trials (RCTs) to assess their true effects. Doctors are being urged, even forced, only to use drugs that have been proved to be valuable by RCTs and similar scientific analyses.

Treatments for heart disease have been the first priority in such evidence-based analyses. Guidelines on them have been issued by authorities such as the British Medical Association, the American College of Physicians and the American Society of Internal Medicine. These august organizations have jointly produced their findings in *Clinical Evidence*, first published in June 1999. They describe it as 'A compendium of the best available evidence for effective health care'.

Although *Clinical Evidence* is intended for practising doctors, it is useful for everyone to know the best practice guidelines for their own condition. Now that doctors and patients are seen as equal partners in the decisions on treatment, it is good for the patients, as well as the doctors, to know what is considered the best treatment for their condition. You can then understand why you, or the person you are caring for, is being treated in a particular way. You may also need help in the hopefully rare case when you or they appear to be getting less than the best attention. The following are the 'key messages' published in *Clinical Evidence* for doctors treating heart disease.

Guidelines on heart attacks

To take a heart attack – a myocardial infarction – first. If you suspect a heart attack, then it is vital to take a whole aspirin tablet immediately. Chew it, then swallow it. There is good evidence that it will work quickly to limit the size and severity of the clot in your coronary artery and limit the damage to your heart muscle. Do it even if you are taking aspirin every day. That's because there's evidence that the heart attack may have started in response to a flood of new platelets flushing out from the bone marrow – and they will not be affected by an aspirin taken an hour or more before. Only a fresh aspirin tablet will deal with them, and stop their clumping together, or to an artery wall, to form a clot.

So it is a good idea to carry an aspirin around with you, just in case. One tablet in a wallet or a handbag is enough. You don't need to have water with it – indeed it is a good idea to chew it, because that will get it into your bloodstream faster. From then on you should take half an aspirin a day for the rest of your life.

The guidelines also make it clear that if you are having a heart attack, the paramedic or doctor who first attends you should give a 'thrombolytic' (streptokinase and/or heparin, or tissue plasminogen activator (tPA) and/or herapin) as soon as possible. This should be combined with a betablocker drug given into a vein to start with, then followed by a betablocker tablet for several years. You should also be given an ACE inhibitor within 24 hours, and continue with it for about a month if you are at a relatively low risk of dying, and for several months if you have any signs of heart failure (the two main ones are breathlessness and ankle swelling). Nitrates are useful to ease symptoms in the early stages after heart attack.

These may seem complicated treatment, but RCTs have proved that all of these treatment steps significantly lower death rates after heart attacks.

If you reach hospital within four hours of the onset of the chest pain, and have the typical ECG changes of poor oxygen flow to the heart muscle (ischaemia), then your chances of survival are greatly improved by having an immediate balloon angioplasty (percutaneous transcoronary angioplasty, or PTCA). If this is done within 90 minutes of reaching hospital by an experienced team in a centre that is regularly performing PTCAs, it will prevent much, and perhaps even all, of the irreversible damage to the heart.

Guidelines on unstable angina

The guidelines on the treatment of unstable angina (see page 82) are equally clear. The most important is that in people who develop unstable angina, starting them on aspirin in a dose of only 325 mg per day (a single standard aspirin tablet) reduces their risk of death from heart attack or stroke by just over a third (35 per cent) over the next six months. The six-month death rates were 14 per cent on placebo and 9 per cent on aspirin, in RCTs involving 4,000 people with unstable angina. Interestingly, although aspirin has a reputation for causing gastric bleeding and upset, it did not do so in these trials.

There was also good evidence that adding the anticoagulant preparations heparin or low molecular weight heparin to aspirin might lower the death rates further, but long-term heparin treatments are complex and may cause bleeding. It is not yet clear that the added advantage over aspirin alone is big enough to be of real clinical benefit. The British and American teams ask for more RCTs on the benefits, or possible disadvantages, of other drugs such as nitrates or betablockers in unstable angina. There is still no hard evidence that performing emergency angioplasty in unstable angina carries advantages over simple treatment with aspirin.

Guidelines on preventing a further heart attack for people who have already had one or more

The biggest problem for anyone who has had a heart attack is how to prevent the next one. This has been extensively covered by many RCTs, the results of which have been reviewed in *Clinical Evidence*. The guidelines run as follows.

'Antiplatelet' treatment, the main one of which is aspirin, 'produces substantial reductions in the risk of serious vascular events' – meaning episodes of unstable angina, heart attacks and strokes. The recommended dose of aspirin is 75 mg per day (a quarter of a standard aspirin), which is as effective as higher doses. In the very few people who are allergic to aspirin, clopidogrel is a safe and effective alternative. Adding anticoagulants gives no advantage over aspirin alone.

The guidelines also recommend betablockers and ACE inhibitors. RCTs have shown that betablockers reduce sudden death rates and death rates from another heart attack in people who have had at least

101

one heart attack before. They also reduce the rate of repeat non-fatal heart attacks.

ACE inhibitors are recommended especially for people with a poorly functioning heart muscle after a heart attack (the medical term for this is left ventricular dysfunction). They help by lowering death rates and the numbers of admissions to hospital for heart failure and for a repeat heart attack. Whether ACE inhibitors should be given to people who have normal heart function after a heart attack is not yet proved.

On the other hand, the guidelines state that many 'anti-arrhythmic' drugs may actually increase the risk of sudden death after heart attack, and advises against them, except in special circumstances. Short-acting calcium channel blockers (those that have to be taken more often than once a day) are not recommended after heart attacks.

In women, although hormone replacement therapy seems to reduce the risks of repeated heart attacks, there is no evidence from the single large RCT that has been published that it actually does so.

Cholesterol lowering with statins, the guidelines state, 'substantially reduces the risk of cardiovascular mortality and morbidity, with no increase in non-cardiovascular mortality'.

Although there is no direct evidence that lowering blood pressure in people with established coronary disease prevents further heart attacks, the guidelines state that the evidence in people with no previous heart 'events' support the need to lower their blood pressure in those at high risk of them. The best evidence for this so far is when betablockers have been used.

Guidelines on non-drug treatments

Much is made in the popular press of the advantages of 'antioxidants' in protecting people against heart attacks. Healthy living, the health columnists keep stressing, must always include eating foods or taking additives that ensure a huge intake of antioxidant compounds such as vitamin E, beta-carotene and vitamin C. Unfortunately there is no proof that this is the case.

Antioxidants, like drugs, have been subject to evidence-based scrutiny by the British and American authorities. The guidelines state that the role of vitamin E, beta-carotene and vitamin C remain unclear.

On the other hand, RCT evidence shows that people who have had coronary thromboses will get substantial benefit from a mediterranean diet that includes plenty of fish, fruit, vegetables, bread, pasta, potatoes, olive oil and rapeseed margarine. On the other hand, RCTs found no benefit from low-fat or high-fibre diets on non-fatal heart attack rates or death rates from heart disease.

The guidelines add that cardiac rehabilitation improves coronary risk factors and reduces the risk of major cardiac events in patients after a heart attack. Many studies (though they are not RCTs) have shown that when people with coronary disease stop smoking they very rapidly reduce their risk of repeated coronary events or death. Nicotine patches, the guidelines state, seem safe in people with coronary disease.

They add that although psychological and stress management may decrease the rates of repeat heart attacks or sudden death in people who have known coronary disease, RCTs that show this are mainly of poor quality.

More recent RCTs comparing medical treatment with coronary artery bypass grafting in people with proven coronary disease show that with modern techniques and the optimal medical treatment, surgery has advantages over medical treatment alone over the next 5 and 10 years. The results of surgery in trials in the 1990s are better than those in the 1980s. Stents are more effective than balloon angioplasty, both in the short and long term.

Appendix 1
Hints to help your heart

This appendix is simply a series of 'rules to live by' if you want to take care of your heart. They are positive, rather than negative – there are few 'thou shalt nots', except for smoking!

– Keep fit. We are built to walk, run, climb and swim: we feel better when we do them. Stay inert and lazy, and we feel worse in the long run, and our hearts complain about it, too.

– Vary your exercise so that you won't be bored. That way, you won't give it up.

– Eat well, of the right foods. Take your proteins in as fish, poultry and cereals, and your fats in vegetable or fish oils. Eat plenty of fruit and enjoy your potatoes baked or boiled in their skins. Eat pastas and rice, and enjoy the different flavours of spices, rather than drown your food in salt. Get to know the wide scope there is for vegetables and fruit. Restrict red meats and dairy products to the occasional treat, and even then cut off the fat.

– Don't worry about your weight: if you are eating correctly and exercising enough, it will look after itself. It will come down, and you will have a new shape to be proud of. Don't go on a diet: you will never stick to it!

– Don't smoke – not even one cigarette a day, If you do, cut them *out*, not down. It is no problem to stop, if you are motivated enough. This book tries to provide the motivation!

– Drink in moderation. That means only on four days a week at most, and no more than three–four standard drinks a day for men and two–three for women. Don't be tempted to backslide on the odd festive occasion – you can enjoy yourself as much sober as drunk – probably a lot more so!

– If a close relative has had a heart attack when relatively young, by all means have your cholesterol checked. If it is high, then change your life so that it comes down. Most people can do this fairly easily – again it depends on your motivation! For those who don't or can't succeed, take advice on cholesterol-lowering drugs.

– Have your blood pressure checked. If it is normal, that is fine. If it is high, discuss how to bring it down into the normal range with your doctor.

– If you have diabetes, keep your blood glucose levels and insulin doses under the best possible control. That can at times be inconvenient, but it may be your best insurance to living longer, with a much healthier heart and circulation.

– If you already have angina, all the advice given above still applies to you. Keep as fit as possible, but do stop and rest when you have the pain. Anyone under 65 with angina should discuss with their doctor the possibility of bypass surgery or angioplasty.

– If your angina seems to be lasting longer than it should, or is more severe than usual – do not hesitate to call for emergency assistance. Fast admission to hospital may be the only way to ensure survival with a good quality of life.

– After a coronary attack, all the rules above apply even more! A heart attack is not a signal to become an invalid, except in very severe cases. Nine out of ten heart attack survivors return to their previous health, and many use their attack as a turning point to a better, happier and healthier lifestyle.

– The new lifestyle is vital to living with a healthy heart: you may add to your chances of a long healthy life by eating three oily fish meals a day. A 75 mg aspirin tablet every day may also help, but you should ask your doctor about that before you start.

No one lives for ever, but if you follow this simple list of rules, you will give yourself more than an even chance of reaching your eighties, and even better, of enjoying them.

Finally, if you are interested in helping heart disease research, then there is one charity that needs your support. The British Heart Foundation:

- funds heart research
- keeps doctors abreast of the latest developments and treatments of heart disease
- provides equipment for specialist hospital heart units and ambulances
- and tries to educate us all on how to take care of our hearts.

If you wish to know more about, or to contribute to, the British Heart Foundation, write to

Broughton House
9 St Mark's Hill
Surbiton
KT6 4SB

The BHF also has ten regional offices throughout Britain, where the staff will be pleased to hear from you. Of all the medical charities, this must be one of the most productive in terms of practical results. I commend it very highly.

Appendix 2
Prescribed drugs for heart disease

This lists the most commonly prescribed drugs for patients with a high risk of atheroma or ischaemic heart disease: they may have been given to help prevent or control angina or an arrhythmia; to prevent a first or subsequent heart attack; or to treat heart failure. The drugs are listed here by their 'generic' names, rather than their trade names. Both names should always be on the label of any prescribed drug. They are grouped according to their action in the body, so that the reason for the prescription should be clear.

Although the drugs in each subgroup have similar overall actions, they do differ among themselves. For any particular patient, one betablocker or calcium antagonist may be preferable to another. The decision must be made on the doctor's assessment of that particular case. This list has been made so that people with heart problems can understand a little more about their own prescriptions: it is *not* intended to recommend any single drug or group of drugs above any other.

Agents to lower risks of angina and heart attack

Hypolipidaemics (lower cholesterol and other blood fats):
  acipimox
  cholestyramine
  colestipol
  bezafibrate
  ciprofibrate
  clofibrate
  fenofibrate
  gemfibrozil
  statins:
    atorvastatin
    cerivastatin
    fluvastatin
    pravastatin
    simvastatin
  eicosapentaenoic acid (EPA)

Anti-anginal agents

Nitrates (reduce the load on the heart, and open areas of poor coronary flow):
  glyceryl trinitrate
  isosorbide dinitrate
  isosorbide mononitrate
  pentaerythritol tetranitrate

Nitrate-like agent
  nicorandil

Betablockers (slow down and lower the force of the heartbeat; may also prevent arrhythmias):
  acebutolol
  atenolol
  bisoprolol
  metoprolol
  nadolol
  oxprenolol
  pindolol
  propranolol
  timolol

Calcium antagonists (reduce the tone and contraction force of heart muscle, open coronary arteries, improving oxygen supply to, and reducing oxygen demand of, heart muscle):
  amlodipine
  diltiazem
  felodipine
  nicardipine
  nifedipine
  nisoldipine
  verapamil

Drugs for acute heart attack

Anticoagulants (prevent further clotting in coronary arteries):
  desirudin
  heparin
  lepirudin

nicoumalone
phenindione
warfarin

Fibrinolytics (break down clot already formed):
alteplase
anistreplase
reteplase
streptokinase
TPA (tissue plasminogen activator)
urokinase

Antiplatelet drugs (prevent clotting arteries):
abciximab
aspirin
clopidrogel
dipyridamole
eptifibatide
tirofiban

Drugs for arrhythmias and heart failure

Anti-arrhythmics (prevent or reverse abnormal heart rhythms):
amiodarone
disopyramide
flecainide
lignocaine
mexiletine
phenytoin
procainamide
propafenone
quinidine
tocainide
Betablockers and calcium antagonists, as described in the anti-angina section, and cardiac glycosides, described below, also have anti-arrhythmic effects.)

Anti-heart failure drugs (help make heart beat stronger and more efficient or reduce load on the heart by lowering resistance in circulation):

ACE inhibitors:
  captopril
  cilazapril
  enalapril
  fosinopril
  lisinopril
  perindopril
  quinapril
  ramipril
  trandolapril
Cardiac glycosides:
  digitalis
  digoxin
'Alpha-blocker':
  prazosin
Diuretics (reduce heart workload by causing excretion of fluid):
  acetazolamide
  amiloride
  bendrofluazide
  bumetanide
  chlorthalidone
  clopamide
  cyclopenthiazide
  ethacrynic acid
  frusemide
  hydrochlorothiazide
  hydroflumethiazide
  methylchlorthiazide
  metolazone
  metyrapone
  piretanide
  polythiazide
  spironolactone
  triamterene
  xipamide

Index